Practical Guide to Paraphilia and Paraphilic Disorders

Richard Balon
Editor

Practical Guide to Paraphilia and Paraphilic Disorders

Springer

Editor
Richard Balon
Department of Psychiatry and Behavioral Neurosciences
Wayne State University
Detroit, MI, USA

Department of Anesthesiology
Wayne State University
Detroit, MI, USA

ISBN 978-3-319-42648-8 ISBN 978-3-319-42650-1 (eBook)
DOI 10.1007/978-3-319-42650-1

Library of Congress Control Number: 2016959001

Printed on acid-free paper

This Springer imprint is published by Springer Nature
The registered company is Springer International Publishing AG
The registered company address is: Gewerbestrasse 11, 6330 Cham, Switzerland

Foreword

Paraphilias/paraphilic disorders are an entity of many unknowns—prevalence, etiology, many treatment and management issues, and others.

This book is intended to be what its title says—a practical, clinically oriented, up-to-date guide to paraphilias/paraphilic disorders. It does not intend to replace some classic or reference volumes such as *Sexual Deviance, Theory, Assessment, and Treatment* [1]. We hope that our volume will serve busy clinicians who may encounter paraphilias/paraphilic disorders and would like to learn some basics about this group of disorders and their management. As this guide is clinically oriented, we have tried to enrich individual chapters by clinical examples wherever appropriate.

To make this book really up-to-date and modern, we included a few topics that are usually not covered in volumes on paraphilias. These include the hotly debated and in the new version of the DSM not yet accepted hypersexual disorder; emerging trends such as online compulsive paraphilic behavior; ethical issues in the management of paraphilic disorders; and cultural aspects of paraphilias/paraphilic disorders.

We also hope that this volume may serve the reader as an introduction to an interesting yet neglected and almost abandoned area of psychiatry.

Richard Balon

Reference

1. Laws DR, O'Donohue WT (eds.) Sexual deviance. Theory, assessment, and treatment. 2nd ed. New York: Guilford; 2008.

Contents

Contributors

Deyadira Baez-Sierra, M.D. Department of Psychiatry and Behavioral Sciences, George Washington University School of Medicine, Virginia Commonwealth University, Inova Fairfax Hospital, Falls Church, VA, USA

Department of Psychiatry, Inova Fairfax Hospital, Falls Church, VA, USA

Chandrika Balgobin, D.O. Department of Psychiatry and Behavioral Sciences, George Washington University School of Medicine, Virginia Commonwealth University, Inova Fairfax Hospital, Falls Church, VA, USA

Richard Balon, M.D. Department of Psychiatry and Behavioral Neurosciences, Wayne State University, Detroit, MI, USA

Department of Anesthesiology, Wayne State University, Detroit, MI, USA

Brad D. Booth, M.D., F.R.C.P.C. Integrated Forensic Program, Division of Forensic Psychiatry, Department of Psychiatry, Royal Ottawa Mental Health Centre, University of Ottawa, Ottawa, ON, Canada,

Peer Briken, M.D., F.E.C.S.M. Institute for Sex Research and Forensic Psychiatry, University Medical Center Hamburg-Eppendorf, Hamburg, Germany

Tara C. Collins, M.D., M.P.H. Department of Psychiatry, University of California, San Francisco, CA, USA

Fritjof von Franqué, Dipl.-Psych., ECPS Institute for Sex Research and Forensic Psychiatry, University Medical Center Hamburg-Eppendorf, Hamburg, Germany

Frederico Duarte Garcia, M.D., Ph.D. Department of Mental Health, Regional Center on Addictions (CRR-UFMG) and Post-graduation in Molecular Medicine of the Federal University of Minas Gerais (UFMG), Belo Horizonte, MG, Brazil

Inserm Unity 1073, Rouen University, Mont-Saint-Aignan, France

David V. Hamilton, M.D., M.A. Department of Psychiatry and Neurobehavioral Sciences, Charlottesville, VA, USA

Waguih William IsHak, M.D., F.A.P.A. Department of Psychiatry and Behavioral Neurosciences, Cedars-Sinai Medical Center, Los Angeles, CA, USA

Christina Tara Khan, M.D., Ph.D. Department of Psychiatry and Behavioral Sciences, Palo Alto, Stanford, CA, USA

National Center for Posttraumatic Stress Disorder, Dissemination and Training Division, Veterans Affairs Palo Alto Health Care System

Julia Machado Khoury, M.D. Department of Mental Health, Regional Center on Addictions (CRR-UFMG) and Post-graduation in Molecular Medicine of the Federal University of Minas Gerais (UFMG), Belo Horizonte, MG, Brazil

Verena Klein, Dipl.-Psych. Institute for Sex Research and Forensic Psychiatry, University Medical Center Hamburg-Eppendorf, Hamburg, Germany

Mário F. Lourenço, M.D., Ph.D. Couple's Clinic, Psychiatric and Mental Health Department, Alto Ave Hospital Center, Guimarães, Portugal

Scott F. Martin, M.D. Department of Psychiatry, Case Western Reserve University School of Medicine, Center for Marital and Sexual Health, Beachwood, OH, USA

A. Pacheco Palha Faculty of Medicine of Porto University, Rua do Carvalho, Porto, Portugal

Laura Weiss Roberts, M.D., M.A. Department of Psychiatry and Behavioral Sciences, Stanford, CA, USA

National Center for Posttraumatic Stress Disorder, Dissemination and Training Division, Veterans Affairs Palo Alto Health Care System

Marco Antônio Valente Roque, M.D. Department of Mental Health, Regional Center on Addictions (CRR-UFMG) and Post-graduation in Molecular Medicine of the Federal University of Minas Gerais (UFMG), Belo Horizonte, MG, Brazil

Jordan Rosen, M.D. Department of Psychiatry and Neurobehavioral Sciences, Charlottesville, VA, USA

Gabriel Tobia, M.D. Department of Psychiatry and Behavioral Neurosciences, Wayne State University, Detroit, MI, USA

Thomas N. Wise, M.D. Department of Psychiatry, Inova Fairfax Hospital, Falls Church, VA, USA

Department of Psychiatry, Johns Hopkins University, Virginia Commonwealth University, George Washington University, Falls Church, VA, USA

Kevan R. Wylie, M.D., F.R.C.P., F.R.C.Psych. Department of Neurosciences, University of Sheffield, Sheffield, South Yorkshire, UK

Rebecca A. Wylie, B.Sc., M.Sc., M.B.Ps.S. Fishawack Facilitate Limited, Brighton, East Sussex, UK

Chapter 1
Introduction to the Realm of Paraphilias

Richard Balon

Paraphilias and what we now call paraphilic disorders have been puzzling, curiosity-arousing, attention attracting, famous and infamous (take masochism and sadism), maligned, and misunderstood for centuries. Our full understanding of paraphilic behaviors is still lacking. The lack of understanding probably starts with the lack of consensus about the definition, its use, and, at times, its, unfortunately, pejorative use.

The term paraphilia is about 100 years old (the introduction of the term is credited to Friedrich Salomon Krauss in 1903, but it was more generally suggested/introduced by Wilhelm Stekel in German in 1908 and later in 1930). Its meaning and definition vary. The word paraphilia is a construction of two Greek words. The first is *para*, the meaning of which could vary from "beside, side by side" to "beyond,

R. Balon, M.D. (✉)
Department of Psychiatry and Behavioral Neurosciences, Wayne State University, Tolan Park Building, 3rd Floor, 3901 Chrysler Service Dr., Detroit, MI 48201, USA

Department of Anesthesiology, Wayne State University, Tolan Park Building, 3rd Floor, 3901 Chrysler Service Dr., Detroit, MI 48201, USA
e-mail: rbalon@wayne.edu

R. Balon (ed.), *Practical Guide to Paraphilia and Paraphilic Disorders*, DOI 10.1007/978-3-319-42650-1_1

past, by" to "abnormal or defective" (e.g., in paranoia) to "irregular, altered." The other term -philia means love, friendship, brotherly love, affection. In "modern" language it could mean a whole spectrum from a friendly feeling toward something or someone, to an abnormal feeling, depending on the context. Thus, paraphilia in a general sense means love beyond the usual (less derogative term) to abnormal love or sexuality (whatever the term normal sexuality means). Some may also define paraphilia as "love for other/marginal object." The term paraphilia was, in a way, meant to replace terms such as sexual deviation, sodomy, or perversion. It seems that this well-meant semantic change has not been really successful. The definition of paraphilic or sexually "deviant" behavior is also problematic from a fuzzy border between the so-called "normal" or acceptable sexual behavior and abnormal sexual behavior. Take the example of occasional mild spanking of one's sexual partner during sexual activity enjoyed and asked for by the partner vs. binding, whipping, and even kicking the sexual partner during sexual activity. Where is the border between acceptable (or normal) behavior and abnormal behavior here?

Diagnosis of Paraphilia/Paraphilic Disorder

As we do not understand the etiology of paraphilias/paraphilic behaviors (like most mental disorders), our definition/diagnosis of paraphilias/paraphilic behaviors is purely descriptive. The Diagnostic and Statistical Manual of Mental Disorders, Fifth Edition (DSM-5) ([1], p 685) states that, "The term *paraphilia* denotes any intense and persistent sexual interest *other than* [Italics mine] sexual interest in genital stimulation or preparatory fondling with phenotypically normal, physiologically mature, consenting human partners. In some instances, the criteria 'intense and persistent' may be difficult to apply, such as in the assessment of persons who are very old or medically ill and who may not have 'intense' sexual interests of any kind. In such circumstances, the term *paraphilia* may be defined as any sexual interest greater than or equal to normophilic sexual interests. There are also specific paraphilias that are generally better described as preferential sexual interests rather than intense sexual interest. Some paraphilias primarily concern the individual's erotic activities, and others concern the individual's erotic target. Examples of the former include intense and persistent interest in spanking, whipping, cutting, binding, or strangulating another person, or an interest in these activities that equals or exceeds the individual's interest in copulation or equivalent interaction with another person. Examples of the latter would include intense or preferential interest in children, corpses, or amputees (as a class), as well as intense or preferential interest in nonhuman animals, such as horses or dogs, or in inanimate objects, such as shoes or articles made of rubber." The DSM-5 also points out a classification scheme for paraphilic disorders, dividing them into two groups: (a) those with anomalous activity preference (these are further divided into *courtship disorders*, which resemble distorted components of human courtship behavior—voyeuristic disorder, exhibitionistic disorder, frotteuristic disorder) and algolagnic disorders, which involve pain and suffering—sexual masochism disorder, sexual sadism disorder); and (b) those with anomalous target preference—one directed at humans (pedophilic disorder) and two directed elsewhere (fetishistic disorder, transvestic disorder) ([1], p 685).

In its attempt to address the wide criticism of labeling paraphilia as mental illness, the DSM-5 introduced the term paraphilic disorder: "*A paraphilic disorder* is paraphilia that is currently causing distress or impairment to the individual or a paraphilia whose satisfaction has entailed personal harm, or risk of harm, to others. A paraphilia is a necessary but not a sufficient condition for having a paraphilic disorder, and a paraphilia by itself does not necessarily justify or require clinical intervention" ([1], pp 685–686) In spite of a wide criticism by many (see below), I view this as an important shift and step in the process of de-pathologizing paraphilias. The previous DSM definitions of paraphilia were basically what the DSM-5 definition of paraphilic disorder is. Paraphilia was a disorder. The DSM-5 recognizes that paraphilia itself is an interest or even behavior which does not necessarily meet the criterion of mental disorder (in the sense of DSM definition of mental disorder). It is important to realize as Paul Fedoroff ([2], p 241) pointed out that paraphilias as a group of disorders are "remarkably consistent in their phenomenology, but highly variable in their expression."

Some have criticized classifying paraphilias/paraphilic disorders as mental illnesses in general terms, opposing what is called the pathologization of nonnormative sexual practices originally called "deviations" or "perversions" [3]. Downing [3] argues that the diagnosis of paraphilic disorder does nothing to overturn what she calls "the conservative and utilitarian view of sexuality as genitally oriented and for reproduction that has colored sexological and psychiatric history" ([3], p 1139). She also argues that using labels such as paraphilia and paraphilic disorder within the psychiatric diagnostic system is more ideological than properly scientific, and that the "normophilic" bias of the DSM is a bias in favor of heteronormativity and reproduction ([2], p 1139). Some (e.g., [4]) have argued that at least some, if not all, paraphilias/paraphilic disorders should not be included in the DSM classification. Shindel and Moser ([4], p 928) suggested that "Evidence-based medicine is now considered the basis of and guide for medical practice. Continuing to include the diagnoses of sexual sadism in the DSM in the absence of empirical evidence to support their inclusion violates a stated principle of the DSM revision process: 'all changes proposed for the text are to be supported by empirical data.' A basic tenet of medicine taught to all physicians is, 'First, do not harm.' These diagnoses have caused harm, been misused, and lack the scientific basis for designating these interests as pathological. The resistance to removing diagnoses which have significant negative effects, no clear positive effects, and no-established utility in patient management is bewildering. Therefore the APA (American Psychiatric Association—mine) should remove sexual masochism and consensual sexual sadism from DSM-5. Based on the same logic, the other non-criminal paraphilias (transvestism, fetishism, partialism) should also be removed. Individuals who engage in non-consensual sexual behavior can (and should) be offered treatment to help them control their sexual urges. Existing psychiatric diagnoses that focus on inability to control behavior can be used. Impulse control maybe a more viable treatment goal than reparative therapies for unusual sexual interests." This is certainly an interesting argument and suggestion, but is it really providing a solution? Most diagnoses in our classification system are not perfect in terms of evidence-based medicine and lack of various empirical data. Should that be a basis for removal of many more diagnoses or should we rather study these behaviors more intensely and comprehensively? Lot has been written about the diagnoses of paraphilia and paraphilic disorder, but as noted by Blanchard [5], the field has not studied the diagnoses of paraphilias/paraphilic disorders properly. He writes that the field trials for DSM-III included three patients with paraphilias. Paraphilias were not included in the field trials for DSM-III-R or for DSM-IV field trials and to my knowledge neither in the DSM-5 field trials. Thus, as Blanchard states, "the sum total of patients who have been studied in conjunction with revising the DSM diagnostic criteria for the paraphilias is 3" ([5], p 861). Thus studying the diagnosis seems to be a better first step than abandoning it.

As pointed out by Moser [6] in his discussion of Ray Blanchard's work, the DSM definition of paraphilia is a definition by concatenation, i.e., by listing things that are paraphilias, yet preferable approach may be a definition by exclusion, i.e., to list everything what is not normophilic. Further issues which the diagnosis of paraphilia and paraphilic disorder faces include the importance of precision in the language defining these disorders and the outside societal and political pressures to define what is "normal," what is "acceptable" for the society and for the forensic arena. For instance, Wakefield [7] pointed out the tension between diagnostic validity and forensic utility of the diagnostic criteria of paraphilias. He noted that, "In order to prevent sexual crimes, 'sexual predator' laws now allow indefinite preventive commitment (at least in the U.S.—mine) of criminals who completed their prison sentences but are judged to have a paraphilic mental disorder that makes them likely to commit another crime. Such proceedings can bypass the usual protections of criminal laws as long as the basis for incarceration is the attribution of a mental disorder. Thus the difficult conceptual distinction between deviant sexual desires that are mental disorders vs. those that are normal variations of sexual preference (even if they are eccentric, repugnant, or illegal if acted upon) has attained important forensic significance. Yet the concept of paraphilic disorders—called 'perversions' in earlier times is inherently fuzzy and controversial and thus open to conceptual abuse for social control purposes" (7 - p 195).

Interestingly, we have been also unable to decide where in our diagnostic systems to classify paraphilias/paraphilic disorders. Previously, the DSM system placed paraphilias under "sexual and gender identity disorders." In the DSM-5, paraphilic disorders are separated from sexual dysfunctions and are placed, almost symbolically, at the very end of the DSM-5, just prior to "Other mental disorders." The International Classification of Diseases (ICD) (in its section on Mental and Behavioral Disorders) classifies paraphilias as "disorders of adult personality and behavior," and among these as "disorders of sexual preference." Sexual dysfunctions, on the other hand, are classified as "behavioral syndromes associated with physiological disturbances and physical factors." The paraphilias listed in ICD-10 include fetishism, fetishistic transvestism, exhibitionism, voyeurism, pedophilia, sadomasochism (sadism, masochism), other disorders of sexual preference (e.g., frotteurism, necrophilia), and disorder of sexual preference not otherwise specified. The DSM classification also lists eight paraphilic disorders (voyeuristic, exhibitionistic, frotteuristic, sexual masochism, sexual sadism, pedophilic, fetishistic, and transvestic—basic classification also used in this book) and all encompassing Other Specified Paraphilic Disorder with examples of what this entity encompasses being telephone scatophilia, necrophilia, zoophilia, coprophilia, klismaphilia, and urophilia. Yet there are several hundreds of described paraphilias in the literature. For instance, Paul Fedoroff lists [8] 111 paraphilias plus paraphilia NOS and Other disorders of sexual preference, from abasiophilia (persistent sexual arousal toward disability) to zoosadism (persistent sexual arousal focused on harm to animals). Milner, Dopke, and Crouch [9] counted more than 150 named paraphilias in both the professional and general literature. However, as they [9] pointed out, many newly named paraphilias appeared to be subtypes of existing paraphilias and thus it is unclear how many newer paraphilias NOS (Not Otherwise Specified) categories or entities are needed ([9], p 390). In their very informative review and descriptions they divide paraphilias NOS to those focused on nonhuman objects (e.g., zoophilia, klismaphilia, mysophilia), suffering or humiliation of oneself or one's partner (e.g., telephone scatophilia, saliromania—soiling or damaging of a partner's clothing or body), children or other nonconsenting persons (e.g., somnophilia, necrophilia), and a large subcategory of those paraphilias having atypical focus involving human subjects (self and others) (e.g., hypoxyphilia, partialism, gerontophilia, or troilism).

There have been other possible paraphilias/paraphilic disorders, some of which were considered for inclusion in DSM-5 (e.g., hypersexual disorder, paraphilic coercive disorder, pedohebephilia, and compulsive online sexual behaviors), some of which are discussed in this book.

Treatment of Paraphilias

Treatment of paraphilias/paraphilic disorders has been a complicated task. General principles are outlined in Chap. 4 of this volume and specific in each chapter devoted to a particular paraphilic disorder. However, there are many unresolved and controversial issues in the management and treatment of paraphilias—now paraphilic disorders. I outlined some of them in the past [10]. These include the question of whether to treat or not to treat and what to treat; goals of treatment; how and with what to treat; length of treatment; possible use of extreme treatments such as castration; and preventive treatment. Another issue is the lack of solid treatment studies.

There is no clear and widely recognized guidance as to whether and when to treat and which paraphilic disorders to treat [10]. Treatment of paraphilic disorders is a minefield of ethical issues, especially when pharmacotherapy is used [11] (some of them are addressed in Chap. 16). The goals of treatment are also not very clear. Should we treat patients to "extinguish" fantasies, or urges, or behaviors? Another ethical question is whose wish and beneficence should we respect, the patient's or society's? The beneficence of society clearly prevails in some paraphilic disorders, such as pedophilic or sadistic ones. But does it prevail in all paraphilic disorders?

We lack data on how long to treat patients with paraphilic disorders. Garcia and Thibault [11] recommend treating severe paraphilias with a high risk of sexual violence for a minimal duration of 3–5 years. They also recommend that mild paraphilias (a bit unclear term) be treated for at least 2 years, then treatment should be discontinued, the patient monitored, and treatment restarted in case of reoccurrence sexual fantasies. However, these recommendations leave many unanswered questions, some of them especially important in the case of paraphilic disorders. As Balon [10] asked: How long should the patient be treated after becoming symptom-free? Should the number of relapses be another guiding principle, similar to the guidance for treatment of depression (three relapses would mean lifelong treatment)—but would society require fewer relapses for starting lifelong treatment of paraphilic disorders?)? Should natural decline of testosterone levels be considered in the hormone treatment of paraphilic disorders?

A preventive approach to paraphilic disorders would probably be quite desirable from the societal point of view and interest. Primary prevention of paraphilic disorders is not possible, as we do not know the etiology of these disorders. Secondary prevention—diagnosing and treating the disorder in its early stages before it causes significant morbidity and harm to others—means quick intervention when the urges, fantasies, and behaviors first occur [10]. That may be problematic as some (probably most) individuals would not seek treatment. It seems impossible to evaluate effectiveness of secondary prevention. Laws [12] proposed that secondary prevention should include targeting children, adolescents, and adults, e.g., make adults aware of unusual sexual activity or interest in children who were abused. Tertiary prevention—reducing the negative effect of the disorder, reducing disorder-related complications, and preventing recurrence is done only in cases of pedophilic disorder, sadism/rape, and exhibitionistic disorder [10]. Again the ethical questions are multiple and guidance regarding treatment length is nonexistent. A solid approach to prevention of paraphilic disorder would probably require creating more programs such as The National Sex Offender Treatment Programme in Canada.

Treatment of paraphilic disorder is also an area of a possible clash between medicine and the legal system. The demands and requirements of the legal system may, and usually are, different. As Borneman [13] pointed out in his book on possible rehabilitation of child molesters, "…if an object of medical treatment, child sex abuse is an illness, and hence requires healing; if an object of law, child sex abuse is an intended crime, and hence deserves punishment. Medicine is about health and illness, law about innocence and guilt. Child sex offenders have become, then, simultaneous or alternating objects of medicine—afflicted by a 'paraphilic disorder'—and of law—individuals who intend to commit or have committed a crime, subjects to the claims of expertise in both fields."

Stigma of Paraphilias/Paraphilic Disorders

As pointed out by Cantor [14], atypical sexual interests remain highly stigmatized in the Western society, especially in the United States. Paraphilic disorders are definitely highly stigmatizing and probably one of the most despised groups of mental disorders (e.g., paraphilic disorder with a sexual interest in prepubescent children—[15]). This stigma limits the acceptance of the individual by the society, the availability of places to live, and, in a way, access to treatment, as individuals suffering from paraphilic disorder usually do not seek treatment on their own and specialized treatments are frequently not available. In some places in the Unites States, being a severe sexual offender (e.g., cases of pedophilic disorder) means basically indefinite if not lifelong sentence. These offenders are, after serving a prison sentence, being held indefinitely in special facilities under a policy of civil commitment, having being deemed "sexually dangerous" or "sexual psychopathic personalities" by courts. The intent is to provide treatment to the most dangerous sex offenders until it is safe for the public for them to go home [16]. Some of them have been held for decades. (In all fairness, these policies are being reevaluated—[16]). As Wakefield ([7], p 196) pointed out, "the Supreme Court (of the United States) has ruled that preventive institutionalization of potential sexual criminals is constitutionally acceptable and does not imply constitutionally barred 'double jeopardy' even after such individuals have served full prison terms for their crimes, but only if it could be demonstrated that the threat of renewed harm upon their release is due to a mental disorder that renders the individual unable to exercise normal-range volitional control over sexual behavior." As discussed before, we do not have the ability to really predict future dangerousness well. As the Court emphasized that dangerousness in the form of inability to control one's impulses must be due to a mental disorder to warrant preventive civil commitment [7], some argued against categorizing paraphilias/paraphilic disorders as mental disorder. Wakefield [7] suggested that diagnostic criteria of paraphilic disorders may be open to forensic abuse. The issue of continuous institutionalization and preventive commitment certainly applies to the individuals who committed severe crimes with harm to others. However, in the public's mind this extends to all paraphilic, or what many call perverse behavior, and thus the stigma expands. The legal definition of what is deviant or paraphilic behavior at times differs from medicine's view of what paraphilic or deviant is. The DSM-5

([1], p 697) criteria of pedophilic disorder note that the person suffering from a pedophilic disorder should be at least age 16 years and at least 5 years older than the child or children with whom he/she is sexually involved. The DSM-5 text also notes that individuals in late adolescence involved in an ongoing sexual relationship with a 12- or 13-year-old should not be included in this diagnostic category. However, there have been many cases of 15–16-year-old boys who after it was revealed that they had sex with girls of the same age or just a bit younger were labeled as sexual offenders and ended-up listed in the Sex Offender Registry.

The stigmatization also impacts other areas of functioning and a person's health. Cruwys and Gunaseelan [17] in a recent survey of depressed patients found that experiencing mental illness (in this case depression) was associated with poorer well-being. However, they also found that social identification magnified, rather than buffered, the relationship between stigma and well-being. Thus, they felt that the stigma of mental illness is a double-edge sword—in addition to the direct harm for well-being, by direct identification with other people suffering from mental illness, stigma might expose sufferers to harmful social influence processes. There is no study like this one in the area of paraphilic disorders, but it could be assumed that the impact of stigma on well-being in patients suffering from paraphilic disorders could be at least the same if not greater. The role of stigma and its impact in paraphilias/paraphilic disorders is underappreciated and needs to be addressed. As Cantor [14] wrote, "anyone with an atypical sexual interest should benefit from greater tolerance." The decrease of stigma or destigmatization of atypical sexual interests or paraphilias/paraphilic disorders is also connected to the issue of civil rights. Here Cantor [14] wrote, "...everyone with atypical sexual interests deserves respect and full recognition of all their civil rights...more importantly, questions of rights fall outside the purview of science. People deserve respect and civil rights *regardless* of the scientific classification of their sexual interest."

Conclusion

The realm of paraphilias/paraphilic disorders is a complicated, poorly understood, stigmatized, and insufficiently studied area. Many conclusions and recommendations about paraphilias/paraphilic disorders have been made based on ideological, philosophical, and political reasoning rather than based on science or clinical observation. Some argue that paraphilias/paraphilic disorders should not be considered disorders and as such should not be classified within our diagnostic system. The arguments came from different points of view, ideological, civil liberties, moral, religious, societal, forensic, or within the profession of psychiatry itself (interestingly, many psychiatrists do not like to take care of difficult or complex patients…and patients with paraphilias/paraphilic disorders are at times difficult, at times complex, and at times both difficult and complex). However, this complexity and involvement of various points of view makes the field of paraphilias more fascinating, intellectually stimulating, and at times therapeutically satisfying.

And, as one of my colleagues once said about another group of not-so-well-liked patients, "at the end, they are still our *patients*." This book is intended to help improve the clinical care of these patients, of course those who feel they need help and seek it.

References

1. American Psychiatric Association. Diagnostic and statistical manual of mental disorders. 5th ed. Arlington: American Psychiatric Association; 2013.
2. Fedoroff JP. Forensic and diagnostic concerns arising from the proposed DSM-5 criteria for paraphilic disorder. J Am Acad Psychiatry Law. 2011;39:238–41.
3. Downing L. Heteronormality and repronormality in sexological "perversion theory" and the DSM-5's "paraphilic disorder" diagnoses. Arch Sex Behav. 2015;44:1139–45.

4. Shindel AW, Moser CA. Why are the paraphilias mental disorders? J Sex Med. 2011;8:927–9.
5. Blanchard R. A brief history of field trials of the DSM diagnostic criteria for paraphilias. Arch Sex Behav. 2011;40:861–2.
6. Moser C. Yet another paraphilia definition fails. Arch Sex Behav. 2011;40:483–5.
7. Wakefield JC. DSM-5 proposed diagnostic criteria for sexual paraphilias: tensions between diagnostic validity and forensic utility. Int J Law Psychiatry. 2011;34:195–209.
8. Fedoroff P. Paraphilic worlds. In: Levine SB, Risen CB, Althof SE, editors. Handbook of clinical sexuality for mental health professionals. 2nd ed. New York: Routledge (Taylor & Francis Group); 2010. p. 401–24.
9. Milner JS, Dopke CA, Crouch JL. Paraphilias not otherwise specified. Psychopathology and theory. In: Laws DR, O'Donohue WT, editors. Sexual deviance. Theory, assessment, and treatment. 2nd ed. New York: Guilford; 2008. p. 394–418.
10. Balon R. Controversies in the diagnosis and treatment of paraphilias. J Sex Marital Ther. 2013;39:7–20.
11. Garcia FD, Thibault F. Current concepts in the pharmacotherapy of paraphilias. Drugs. 2011;71:771–90.
12. Laws DR. The public health approach. A way forward? In: Laws DR, O'Donohue WT, editors. Sexual deviance. Theory, assessment, and treatment. 2nd ed. New York: Guilford; 2008. p. 611–28.
13. Borneman J. Cruel attachments. The ritual rehab of child molesters in Germany. Chicago: The University of Chicago Press; 2015. p. 58.
14. Cantor JM. Is homosexuality a paraphilia? The evidence for and against it. Arch Sex Behav. 2012;41:237–47.
15. Jahnke S, Schmidt AF, Geradt M, Hoyer J. Stigma-related stress and its correlates among men with pedophilic sexual interest. Arch Sex Behav. 2015;44:2173–87.
16. Davey M. Freedom eludes sex offenders after prison. Int NY Times. 2015:1 + 4.
17. Cruwys T, Gunaseelan S. "Depression is who I am": mental illness identity, stigma and wellbeing. J Affect Disord. 2016;189:36–42.

Recommended Reading

Laws DR, O'Donohue WT, editors. Sexual deviance. Theory, assessment, and treatment. 2nd ed. New York: Guilford; 2008.
Hicky EW, editor. Sex crimes and paraphilia. Upper Saddle River: Prentice-Hall Publisher; 2005.

Chapter 2
General Information: History, Etiology and Theory (e.g., Courtship), Diagnosis, Comorbidity and Prevalence

Richard Balon

Historical Perspective

The descriptions of what we call paraphilias or paraphilic behaviors appear in various texts and pictorial art since the ancient times. Some old cave paintings picture men having sex with animals. One of the oldest texts mentioning paraphilic behavior is the Bible, as pointed out by Aggrawal [1]. We also know that some paraphilia, e.g., pedophilia and hebephilia, or what some would call pedohebephilia, were fairly benevolently practiced in Ancient Greece and Old Rome. What we now call paraphilias and paraphilic disorders were called by different names and terms by various societies, e.g., sexual deviation, perversion, bestiality, and others. Individual sexual deviations (now paraphilias/paraphilic disorders) have

---

R. Balon, M.D. (✉)
Department of Psychiatry and Behavioral Neurosciences, Wayne State University, Tolan Park Building, 3rd Floor, 3901 Chrysler Service Dr., Detroit, MI 48201, USA

Department of Anesthesiology, Wayne State University, Tolan Park Building, 3rd Floor, 3901 Chrysler Service Dr., Detroit, MI 48201, USA
e-mail: rbalon@wayne.edu

R. Balon (ed.), *Practical Guide to Paraphilia and Paraphilic Disorders*, DOI 10.1007/978-3-319-42650-1_2

been described in different texts, starting with the Bible (here, e.g., voyeurism, bestiality, exhibitionism, necrophilia-1). A couple of the individual paraphilia names (sadism and masochism) came from the description in fiction literature. The term sadism originated with Marquis Donatien Alphonse Francois de Sade, a French nobleman and sexual libertine, who practiced and described in his novellas and other writings various "deviant" sexual practices, including what we call sadism or sadistic practices. Interestingly, de Sade was institutionalized in "lunatic asylums" several times and died in one, where he had what we would call a pedophilic relationship till his death. Masochism is called after an Austrian nobleman Baron Leopold von Sacher-Masoch who also practiced various what we would call paraphilic behaviors (including masochism) and described masochism in his story of *Venus in Furs*. Interestingly, von Sacher-Masoch was also under psychiatric care in his late life and some even claim that he died in an asylum (unconfirmed). The term masochism was introduced into medical terminology by Austrian psychiatrist/sexologist Richard Freiherr von Krafft-Ebing in his famous book *Psychopathia Sexualis* (first published in 1886).

Medicine, psychiatry, and psychoanalysis have gradually become more interested in sexual deviations and, over the last century or so, have attempted to explain their origins and find treatment. Psychoanalysts, starting with Sigmund Freud, have presented many interesting cases and their psychoanalytic interpretations, but unfortunately have not been successful either in improving our understanding of sexual deviations or in finding effective treatments. The attention has gradually shifted to attempts to identify biological causes and treatments. The entertained underlying causes of sexual deviances have ranged from poor impulse control to obsessive compulsive spectrum disorders and personality disorders. The main change has been the conceptualization of sexual deviance or paraphilia as a medical condition rather than a matter of choice or lifestyle.

Though the term paraphilia was around for many years of the last century, it entered the Diagnostic and Statistical

Manual of Mental Disorders (DSM) only in its third edition, DSM-III [2], where paraphilias were included in the section on Psychosexual Disorders. Previous editions used the term sexual deviation and classified them under personality disorder of sociopathic subtype (DSM-I) or under personality disorders and certain other nonpsychotic mental disorders (DSM-II). Interestingly, the notion of classifying paraphilias as personality disorders is kept in the ICD classification, where paraphilias are included under disorders of adult personality and behavior, and among them as "disorders of sexual preference." As the DSM-III [2] became more descriptively specific, it described that the essential features of paraphilias was unusual or bizarre imagery or acts that are necessary for sexual excitement ([2], p 266). It also required that "Such imagery or acts tend to be insistently and involuntarily repetitive and generally involve either: (1) preference for use of a nonhuman object for sexual arousal, (2) repetitive sexual activity with humans involving real or simulated suffering or humiliation, or (3) repetitive sexual activity with nonconsenting partners ([2], p 266). Interestingly, the specific paraphilias listed in DSM-III do not match the list of specific paraphilic disorders included in DSM-5 [3]. They (DSM-III) include fetishism, transvestism, zoophilia, pedophilia, exhibitionism, voyeurism, sexual masochism, and sexual sadism (DSM-5 does not include zoophilia among specific paraphilic disorders, but includes frotteuristic disorder as one of the main paraphilic disorders)."

The selection of specific paraphilic disorders for inclusion in the classification and diagnostic manuals is based, as pointed out in DSM-5 ([3], p 685), on two main reasons, "… they are relatively common, in relation to other paraphilic disorders; and some of them entail actions for their satisfaction that, because of their noxiousness or potential harm to others, are classed as criminal offenses" ([1], p 685). The former reasoning is interesting, as we really do not know much about the prevalence of paraphilic disorders (see below), and the prevalence could be impacted by cultural (see Chap. 18) and other issues. As Gordon [4] noted, "Whilst it is almost certainly the case that all human societies through history have imposed limits on the types of sexual behavior regarded as acceptable, a degree of variation across cultures has occurred, whilst, within cultural traditions, change in sexual mores may occur over time. Throughout history, it is evident that societies require a concept of sexual deviancy, but that it is subject to changes in social perspectives. Religious interest tends to be more associated with moral condemnation of sexual deviance and the secular with greater liberalism" ([4], p 79). The latter reason for inclusion in the DSM ("noxiousness" and potential harm to others) seems a bit more plausible. The selection of several specific paraphilias/paraphilic disorders also does not emphasize enough the fact that persons suffering from a paraphilia/paraphilic disorder usually suffer from more than one paraphilia/paraphilic disorder [5].

The treatment approaches to paraphilias have developed over the last century or two. Many persons suffering from paraphilias/paraphilic disorders were institutionalized in asylums, either for the lack of treatment, or comorbidity with other mental disorders, or because the society simply did not know what to do and how to prevent harm to others (e.g., in cases of pedophilia and sadism). However, starting in the 1960s, the asylums gradually emptied and disappeared, due to the availability of new medications for the mentally ill and due to the extension of civil rights movement to the mentally ill. However, as pointed out by Booth and Gulati [6] and others, for a large number of mentally ill the release from asylums meant the lack of appropriate community support and appropriate supervision. Many of these individuals then migrated into the criminal justice system as part of "transinstitutionalization" ([6], p 184). The number of asylum institutionalized mentally ill decreased while the number of mental illness among inmates increased inversely. The same has happened in the case of sexual offenders who have been previously institutionalized in asylums. It is not clear whether the transinstitutionalization of sexual offenders in any way contributed to efforts to find new treatments for paraphilias/paraphilic disorders.

The individual, mostly psychodynamic psychotherapy, for various paraphilias was frequently quite interesting in various interpretations of paraphilias, but hardly applicable for use in the general population of individuals suffering from paraphilias/paraphilic disorders. Behavioral and other therapies for paraphilias started to be used in the 1960s. Aversive therapy was abandoned fairly quickly, mostly for ethical reasons. Other therapies, such as cognitive-behavioral (CBT), were gradually introduced and CBT has become a mainstay ingredient in the treatment of paraphilias/paraphilic disorders. For a long time, the Relapse Prevention Model dominated the area of psychological treatments for sexual offenders. However, the effectiveness of this model remains controversial [7]. More recently, other approaches, such as the Good Lives Model [8] and Motivational Interviewing, were introduced into integrated comprehensive treatment models of paraphilias/paraphilic disorders. It is quite difficult to evaluate the effectiveness of many programs using psychological treatments in the outpatient settings where most psychiatrists see patients with paraphilias/paraphilic disorders, as these programs are usually designed for sex offenders and available in correctional facilities.

Biological, or more correctly what has been called biological, treatment of paraphilias started with surgical castration in the late 1800s, though as Scott and Holmberg [9] pointed out, surgical castration has been used as a means of social control (eunuchs, castrati) for centuries. However, with the advent of modern hormonal therapy and psychopharmacology, and also due to the civil rights groups lobbying, the use of surgical castration was gradually replaced by what is called chemical castration. Various hormones were prescribed to males with paraphilias to curb their deviant or paraphilic behavior by either blocking androgens or administering antiandrogens. Estrogens, such as diethylstilbestrol and progesteronal compounds, were prescribed originally. However, as they had unpleasant side effects (including possible breast carcinoma), their use had been limited. They were replaced by other, mostly injectable preparations which either block androgens or are antiandrogens. Medroxyprogesterone acetate (MPA) started to be used in the United States during the 1960s to diminish sexual fantasies and decrease sexual impulses [9]. MPA induces testosterone reductase in the liver and thus reduces the levels of circulating testosterone, and also blocks follicle stimulation hormone and luteinizing hormone. It is not a true antiandrogen, as it does not compete with antiandrogens at the androgen receptor level. Later on, other hormonal preparations, including cyproterone acetate (true antiandrogen, not available in the USA), leuprolide acetate, triptorelin, flutamide, nilutamide (example of nonsteroidal, pure antiandrogen), and goserelin acetate (used also in the treatment of male-to-female transsexuals) have been introduced.

Other, nonhormonal preparations started to be used for management of paraphilias, especially those paraphilias not considered highly dangerous, for various reasons. The main reasons include serious unpleasant side effects of hormonal preparations, various ethical and legal [9] challenges to "chemical castration," anti-dopamine activities of some medications (dopamine is viewed as a neurotransmitter of reward/excitement, including sexual excitement), and a view/observation of some clinicians and researcher that paraphilias are part of the obsessive-compulsive spectrum (obsessions are similar to sexual fantasies, both paraphilic and nonparaphilic; and compulsive behavior could be non-paraphilic and paraphilic). Various antipsychotics (e.g., fluphenazine enanthate [not available in the USA], benperidol, chlorpromazine, clozapine, and risperidol) have been occasionally used with various successes. The use of older antipsychotics has become more restricted because of the tardive dyskinesia risk. There are almost no reports on the use of newer antipsychotics in this indication. On the other hand, serotonergic antidepressants (selective serotonin reuptake inhibitors and the tricyclic antidepressant clomipramine) have been studied and used relatively frequently [10]. The use of serotonergic antidepressants in paraphilias was based on the phenomenological similarity of paraphilias and obsessive-compulsive and impulse control disorders and the efficacy of serotonergic drugs in these disorders. Some of the side effects of serotonergic drugs (decreased libido and delayed ejaculation/anorgasmia) have probably also played a role in some clinicians' decision to use them.

Anecdotally, some other psychotropic medications (such as buspirone and mood stabilizers) have also been used in the management of paraphilias/paraphilic disorders.

Historically, most biological treatments of paraphilias/paraphilic disorders have been developed based on either theories about of what may play a role in the expression of paraphilias/paraphilic disorders (hormones, antipsychotics), or on serendipitous observations. Unfortunately, we will probably not see any development of new treatments for paraphilias/paraphilic disorder for the following reasons [11]:

(a) Paraphilias/paraphilic disorders are rare, thus it is difficult to get a large and homogenous enough study sample.
(b) Paraphilias/paraphilic disorders are not socially acceptable, and individuals suffering from them (or sex offenders) usually do not seek treatment voluntarily.
(c) Comorbidity rates, especially for personality disorders and substance abuse, among serious offenders, are high.
(d) Ethical considerations frequently do not allow for double-blind placebo-controlled trials, especially with violent offenders.

Etiology

The etiology of paraphilias/paraphilic disorders is unknown. Various interesting theories on their etiology have been postulated through the last century or so. As noted before, psychoanalysts starting with Sigmund Freud (who coined terms such as polymorphous perversity, or scoptophilia) have analyzed various individual cases, but like many others, have not provided a cohesive and comprehensive "general" theory of paraphilias. Also, there are no empirical data demonstrating the effectiveness of psychodynamic psychotherapy in paraphilias beyond individual developmental issues.

Some interesting theories and hypotheses were developed by John Money and Kurt Freund. John Money (e.g., [12]) proposed an explanatory theory of paraphilias using the concept of "lovemaps." His theory suggests that though human beings are genetically programmed, there are developmental or critical periods during which various sexual interests develop. He compared it to the development or acquisition of one's language—the child has a potential to develop any spoken language, but the language the child ultimately speaks is determined by the early life environment and experience. According to Money lovemaps are not present at birth, but develop shortly after birth and usually fully manifest in puberty or even later, at times triggered by some relevant experience. He proposed heterosexual, homosexual, vandalized, and paraphilic lovemaps. According to his theory, paraphilic lovemaps include forbidden, ridiculed, socially unacceptable sexual fantasies. Paraphilic lovemaps could develop by "vandalizing" the ordinary lovemap by sexual abuse, or could arise from nonsexual yet genitally arousing experience in a child.

Kurt Freund (e.g., [13, 14]) argued that voyeurism, exhibitionism, frotteurism, obscene telephone calling, and preferential rape (not included in any diagnostic classification) can be viewed as expressions of a disturbance in a common regulatory system. These expressions can be viewed as distortions of the normal courtship process in males. "The term 'courtship' is taken from the ethological literature, and refers to the sequence of dyadic behavioral interactions that precede and initiate sexual intercourse…The reference system…involves four phases; (1) a finding phase, consisting of locating and appraising a potential partner; (2) an affiliative phase, characterized by nonverbal and verbal overtures such as looking, smiling, and talking to potential partner; (3) a tactile phase, in which physical contact is made; and (4) a copulatory phase, in which sexual intercourse occurs….voyeurism can be viewed as a distortion of the finding phase, exhibitionism as a distortion of the affiliative phase, frotteurism as a distortion of the tactile phase, and rape as a distortion of the copulatory phase" [14]. Freund's courtship theory provides a fairly coherent developmental explanation of some, but not all paraphilias/paraphilic disorders.

Biologically oriented research has also failed to bring much insight into paraphilias/paraphilic disorders. As summarized by Krueger and Kaplan [15], there are no abnormalities in endocrinological functioning in paraphilias, except for one study showing increased responsiveness of luteinizing hormone to infusion of luteinizing hormone releasing hormone in a group of pedophilic subjects. Jordan and colleagues [16] reviewed the literature on the role of testosterone in sexuality and paraphilias and concluded that there appears to be a sex-steroid-related genetic influence on antisocial traits, externalizing behavior, and sexual behavior. Maybe it is the first step pointing in the right direction, yet these conclusions are preliminary. Similarly, imaging studies data have not been very helpful so far. The results of these studies are mixed, with some studies reporting neuropsychological and brain imaging abnormalities in individuals with a history of child molestation and/or paraphilias compared with controls while others do not [15].

Interestingly, paraphilic behaviors have been described in many cases of traumatic brain injury, epilepsy, stroke, dementia, Tourette's syndrome, and Parkinson's disease. The occurrence of paraphilias or paraphilic behavior in patients with Parkinson's disease points in an interesting causative direction. According to Solla and colleagues [17], although the evidence on paraphilia in Parkinson's disease patients remains anecdotal, available data point to these phenomena as likely sequelae of high-dose dopaminomimetic treatment and, accordingly, the intensity of paraphilic urges is typically attenuated by the reduction of dopaminomimetic doses, sometimes in association with atypical antipsychotics. Solla and colleagues [17] actually recommend to routinely ask Parkinson's disease patients about paraphilias. The dopaminergic involvement would support Kafka's tenuous monoamine hypothesis of paraphilias [18].

Diagnosis

As noted in Chap. 1, the diagnostic criteria of paraphilias/paraphilic disorders developed over the last century have become more descriptive and specific, especially in the DSM system. However, as noted, these criteria are specific only for what are believed to be the most common eight paraphilic disorders. Neither the DSM-5 [3] nor any other diagnostic system really captures the richness of paraphilic pathology in its wide spectrum.

Each specific paraphilic disorder has at least two main criteria (Voyeuristic, Pedophilic, and Fetishistic disorder each have a third, more specific diagnostic criterion): Criterion A, which specifies the qualitative nature of the paraphilia, and Criterion B, which specifies the negative consequences of the paraphilia (mostly distress, but also harm to others). As the DSM-5 points out ([3], p 686) the term diagnosis of paraphilic disorder should be reserved for individuals who meet both Criterion A and Criterion B. If an individual meets only Criterion A, he or she should be said to have that specific paraphilia described in Criterion A, but not a paraphilic disorder. Most paraphilic disorders have also attached specifiers—actually seven of them "In a controlled environment" and "In full remission" specifiers (pedophilic disorder does not have these two specifiers), and some have further specifiers (see each particular paraphilic disorder chapter).

The huge area of the rest of paraphilic disorders (presumably less-frequent ones) is covered under the diagnostic category of Other Specified Paraphilic Disorder. These disorders (e.g., Klismaphilic disorder, Necrophilic disorder) should also have their psychopathology present for at least 6 months and should cause marked distress or impairment in social, occupational, or other important areas of functioning ([3], p 705), or harm to oneself or others (mine) to be labeled paraphilic *disorders*. Other paraphilic disorders can be also specified as in remission and/or as occurring in a controlled environment ([3], p 705).

The severity/strength assessment of paraphilias/paraphilic disorders is left to the clinician. As suggested by the DSM-5 ([3], p 686), in a clinical interview or in a self-administered questionnaire, patients can be asked whether their fantasies, urges, or behaviors are weaker, same as usual, or stronger. Specialists in this area may use more psychophysiological tests of sexual interest, such as phaloplethysmography in males and viewing time in males and females.

An important note: As pointed out by Krueger and Kaplan ([15], p 393): "...there is a difference between the term 'paraphilia' and 'sex offender.' 'Sex offender' is a legal term, whereas the term 'paraphilia' denotes a sexual disorder according to the DSM-IV [mine: and according to the DSM-5]. No all sex offenders have paraphilias."

Comorbidity

Paraphilias/paraphilic disorders are frequently comorbid with other disorders or conditions. Comorbidity of paraphilias/paraphilic disorders with another paraphilia/paraphilic disorders is common. Examples include frequent comorbidity of "courtship" disorders—voyeuristic, exhibitionistic, and frotteuristic with each other, or co-occurrence of fetishism with masochism, or transvestism with autoerotic asphyxia.

Paraphilia/paraphilic disorders are also comorbid with other mental disorders, namely with personality disorders (e.g., antisocial personality disorder in some paraphilias/paraphilic disorders, especially those associated with harm to others; also, as noted, some classification systems include paraphilias in the category of disorders of adult personality and behavior) and substance-related and addictive disorders. Paraphilias/paraphilic disorders are also frequently comorbid with hypersexuality (addressed in Chap. 14). Other frequently comorbid disorders and conditions include mood disorders (both depressive and bipolar), anxiety disorders, attention-deficit hyperactivity disorder, and conduct disorder in youths.

Prevalence

The prevalence and incidence of paraphilias/paraphilic disorders is unknown. As Fedoroff wrote [19], the question about prevalence or incidence of paraphilia/paraphilic disorders is "…unanswerable, since any survey must deal with the fact that people are highly reluctant to disclose unconventional sexual interests, especially to surveyors." Krueger and Kaplan [15] voiced a similar opinion pointing out that many of the paraphilic behaviors are illegal and some are subject to mandatory reporting in the United States and many other countries. They noted that questions about paraphilias and paraphilic behavior were not included in national epidemiological surveys of mental disorders. The prevalence of paraphilias/paraphilic disorders may only be inferred from indirect evidence [15]. Most authors (note, not studies) suggest prevalence of 1 % of general population, but they, as Fedoroff [19] suggests, actually mean 1 % of the adult male population. Paraphilias/paraphilic disorders are predominantly disorders of men with the exception of masochistic disorder.

The DSM-5 [3] mentions some prevalence numbers for specific paraphilias/paraphilic disorders. These numbers are drawn from different sources as follows: the highest possible lifetime prevalence for voyeuristic disorder is approximately 12 % in males and 4 % in females (p 688); highest possible prevalence for exhibitionistic disorder in the male population is approximately 2–4 % (p 690); frotteuristic acts may occur in up to 30 % of adult males in the general population and approximately 10–14 % of adult males seen in the outpatient settings for paraphilic disorders and hypersexuality have a presentation that meets the diagnostic criteria for frotteuristic disorders (p 692–693); in Australia, it has been estimated that 2.2 % of males and 1.3 % of females had been involved in bondage and discipline, sadomasochism, or dominance and submission in the past 12 months (p 694). Depending on the criteria for sexual sadism, the prevalence of sadism/sadistic disorder varies widely, from 25 to 30 % (!-mine) and among civilly committed offenders in the United States less than 10 % have sexual sadism, and among individuals who have committed sexually motivated homicides, rates of sexual sadism disorder range from 37 to 75 % (p 696). The highest possible prevalence for pedophilic disorder in the male population is approximately 3–5 %, the prevalence of pedophilic disorder in females is even more uncertain and likely a small fraction of the prevalence in males (p 698). No prevalence for fetishistic disorder is mentioned in DSM-5. Transvestic disorder is rare in males and extremely rare in females, fewer than 3 % of males report having ever been sexually aroused by dressing in women's attire (p 703). Nothing is known about the prevalence of the other more than 100 paraphilias/paraphilic disorders. These numbers only emphasize how little we really know about the prevalence of paraphilias/paraphilic disorders (not to mention the incidence).

I agree with Fedoroff [19] that paraphilias/paraphilic disorders are far more prevalent than 1 % (at least some practices of paraphilic behavior) and that the prevalence fluctuates. Judging from some cyberspace subcultures, some paraphilic behaviors are probably much more frequent than we think. Fedoroff [19] also believes that we are now able to offer treatments that can change the rate of paraphilic disorders ([19], p 408). Importantly, the rates of paraphilias/paraphilic disorders may also vary in different cultures (we really do not know) and are impacted by cultures, cultural practices, and perceptions.

Conclusion

Paraphilias/paraphilic disorders have been a puzzling part of psychiatry and sexuology practically since the inceptions of these disciplines. There are many theories on their etiology, yet as in almost all mental disorders, the etiology remains unknown and is probably multifactorial. Paraphilias/paraphilic disorders are frequently comorbid with other paraphilias/paraphilic disorders and with substance use disorders and personality disorders and many other mental and also neurological disorders. The prevalence of paraphilias is unknown, estimated to be around 1 % of the general population or higher. Paraphilias/paraphilic disorders are predominantly disorders of men with the exception of masochistic disorder (though we do not know much about the prevalence and gender distribution of most of the less-frequent paraphilias/ paraphilic disorders).

References

1. Aggrawal A. References to the paraphilias and sexual crimes in the Bible. J Forensic Leg Med. 2009;16:109–14.
2. American Psychiatric Association. Diagnostic and statistical manual of mental disorders. 3rd ed. Washington, DC: American Psychiatric Association; 1980.
3. American Psychiatric Association. Diagnostic and statistical manual of mental disorders. 5th ed. Arlington: American Psychiatric Association; 2013.
4. Gordon H. The treatment of paraphilias: an historical perspective. Crim Behav Ment Health. 2008;18:79–87.
5. Bradford JM, Boulet J, Pawlak A. The paraphilias: a multiplicity of deviant behaviours. Can J Psychiatry. 1992;37:104–8.
6. Booth BD, Gulati S. Mental illness and sexual offending. In: Bradford JMW, Ahmed AG (Eds.): Sexual deviation and treatment. Psychiatr Clin North Am. 2014;37:183–94.
7. Marshall WL, Marshall LE. Psychological treatments of sex offenders. Recent innovations. In: Bradford JMW, Ahmed AG (Eds.): Sexual deviation and treatment. Psychiatr Clin North Am. 2014;37:163–71.
8. Willis GM, Ward T, Levenson JS. The good lives model (GLM): an evaluation of GLM operationalization in North American treatment programs. Sex Abuse. 2014;26:58–81.
9. Scott CL, Holmberg T. Castration of sex offenders: prisoners' rights versus public safety. J Am Acad Psychiatry Law. 2003;31:502–9.
10. Balon R. Pharmacological treatment of paraphilias with focus on antidepressants. J Sex Marital Ther. 1998;24:241–54.
11. Segraves RT, Balon R. Sexual pharmacology. Fast facts. New York: WW Norton; 2003. p. 288.

12. Money J. Paraphilias: phenomenology and classification. Am J Psychother. 1984;38:164–79.
13. Freund K, Watson R. Mapping the boundaries of courtship disorder. J Sex Res. 1990;27:589–606.
14. Freund K, Seto MC. Preferential rape in the theory of courtship disorder. Arch Sex Behav. 1998;27:433–43.
15. Krueger RB, Kaplan MG. The paraphilic and hypersexual disorders: an overview. J Psychiatr Pract. 2001;7:391–403.
16. Jordan K, Fromberger P, Stolpmann G, Muller JL. The role of testosterone in sexuality and paraphilia—a neurobiological approach. Part II: testosterone and paraphilia. J Sex Med. 2011;8:3008–29.
17. Solla P, Bortolato P, Cannas A, Mulas CS, Marrosu F. Paraphilias and paraphilic disorders in Parkinson's disease: a systematic review of literature. Mov Disord. 2015;30:604–13.
18. Kafka MP. A monoamine hypothesis for the pathophysiology of paraphilic disorder. Arch Sex Behav. 1997;26:343–58.
19. Fedoroff P. Paraphilic worlds. In: Levine SB, Risen CB, Althof SE, editors. Handbook of clinical sexuality for mental health professionals. 2nd ed. New York: Routledge (Taylor & Francis Group); 2010. p. 401–24.

Chapter 3
Assessment and Basic Management Principles of Paraphilic Disorders

Deyadira Baez-Sierra, Chandrika Balgobin, and Thomas N. Wise

Paraphilias vs. Paraphilic Disorders

The word paraphilia comes from the Greek word *para*, which means deviation, and *philia*, which means beyond usual love or attraction. The DSM-IV TR classifies paraphilias within the Sexual and Gender Identity disorders and defines them

---

Portion of this chapter are modified parts of a chapter previously published in a chapter of Clinical Manual of Sexual Disorders edited by Richard Balon, Robert Taylor Segraves, Chapter: Paraphilic Disorders, Authors: Jeanne M. Lackamp, M.D., Cynthia Osborne, MSW, Thomas N. Wise, M.D., pages 335–370. It has been revised to reflect new data.

D. Baez-Sierra, M.D.
Department of Psychiatry and Behavioral Sciences, George Washington University School of Medicine, Virginia Commonwealth University, Inova Fairfax Hospital, 3300 Gallows Road, Falls Church, VA 22042, USA

Department of Psychiatry, Inova Fairfax Hospital, 3300 Gallows Road, Falls Church, VA 22042, USA

C. Balgobin, D.O.
Department of Psychiatry and Behavioral Sciences, George Washington University School of Medicine, Virginia Commonwealth University, Inova Fairfax Hospital, 3300 Gallows Road, Falls Church, VA 22042, USA

R. Balon (ed.), *Practical Guide to Paraphilia and Paraphilic Disorders*, DOI 10.1007/978-3-319-42650-1_3

by recurrent intense, sexually arousing fantasies, sexual urges, or behaviors involving nonhuman objects, the suffering or humiliation of oneself or one's partner or children or nonconsenting persons that occur over a period of 6 months which cause clinically significant distress or impairment in social, occupational, or other important areas of functioning. Paraphilias listed on the DSM-IV TR includes exhibitionism, frotteurism, fetishism, pedophilia, sexual masochism sexual sadism, transvestic fetishism, and voyeurism [1].

The DSM-5 implemented various changes, in regard to the classification of the paraphilic urges, behaviors, and fantasies which includes eliminating the paraphilic behavior from the sexual and gender identity category and renaming it to its own category and establishing a difference between paraphilias and paraphilic disorder, the elimination of paraphilic disorder NOS, the addition of other specified paraphilic disorder and unspecified paraphilic disorder. The DSM-5 defines a paraphilia as any intense and persistent sexual interest other than genital stimulation, or preparatory fondling between phenotypically normal, physically mature, consenting human partners. Paraphilias may be indicative of sexual interest greater than or equal to normophilic sexual interests [2].

The criterion A for paraphilic disorders is defined as intense, recurrent sexual arousal that occurs over the period of 6 months. The Criterion B requires the person acting upon sexual urges with nonconsenting victims, i.e., voyeuristic disorder, exhibitionist disorder, frotteuristic disorder, and sexual sadism disorder, and has caused clinically significant distress or impairment in social occupational setting or other areas of

T.N. Wise, M.D. (✉)
Department of Psychiatry, Inova Fairfax Hospital,
3300 Gallows Road, Falls Church, VA 22042, USA

Department of Psychiatry, Johns Hopkins University, Virginia Commonwealth University, George Washington University,
3300 Gallows Road, Falls Church, VA 22042, USA
e-mail: Thomas.Wise@inova.org

functioning. The diagnosis of paraphilic disorder can be made if both Criterions A and B are met, thus the major differences between paraphilia and paraphilic disorder are the negative consequences of the behavior, including distress, impairment, or harm to others. Nevertheless, in pedophilic disorder, the element of the nonconsenting victim was not included. The newly added criterion C requires a minimum age of 18 years old for the diagnosis of voyeuristic disorder. Also, two new course specifiers were added; in full remission, 5-year duration and in a controlled environment (with the exception of pedophilia) [2].

The DSM-5 paraphilic disorders have been criticized due to problems with definition by exclusion, which pathologizes non-genital sexual arousal or sexual practices of consenting adults like sexual masochism, fetishistic disorder, and transvestic disorder, thus potentially increasing the false positives [3]. Another limitation with the DSM-5 definition is that it is based on culturally or individually specific criteria, minimizes the problems of non-consent (especially with pedophilic disorder) and there are a lack of field trials [4] and there is limited empirical data based on paraphilias. An additional issue with the new definition has to do with the interpretation of the DSM-5 in forensic settings. For example, an individual could be identified as having a paraphilic disorder based on sexual behavior, without taking into consideration the paraphilic arousal pattern [3] or the etiology of that behavior (substance-induced, frontal lobe injury, developmental disability, manic episode, neurodegenerative disorder), which could also lead to an increase in the false negatives [5]. In contrast, there are studies that show sexually criminal behavior unrelated to the sexual arousal pattern [6].

Assessment of Paraphilic Disorders

Evaluation of paraphilias includes a comprehensive examination including interview, sexual history, questionnaires, collateral information from records or informants, screening for comorbid psychiatric disorders, and self-report. The first step involves getting informed consent from the patient, alerting him that the evaluative process may prove stressful, and advising him of the necessary limits of confidentiality regarding current or potential abuse situations. Patients should know that clinicians will be obligated to report information disclosed during clinical interviews, if "mandatory reporting" requirements apply [7]. While this may have an impact on the completeness of patients' disclosures to their clinicians during treatment, knowing state law and being able to communicate this clearly to patients during the initial evaluation is essential. The clinician must present him- or herself as willing to discuss patients' sexual issues openly. While it is the clinician's goal to establish rapport and to be receptive to sensitive material from any patient (particularly since many general psychiatric patients have sexual concerns and/or experience sexual side effects from medications), it is pivotal in this patient population. It is also important to remember that patients may habitually minimize or deny problematic behaviors, and may have significant cognitive distortions upon which they rely for rationalizing their behavior [8, 9].

Instead of focusing immediately on current paraphilic material, clinicians should start by inquiring about the patient's complete sexual history—paraphilic issues, non-paraphilic issues, childhood sexual experiences or activities, adult sexual experiences or activities, or lack thereof. This will help provide the clinician with appropriate background, instead of targeting paraphilic issues in isolation [10]. As noted earlier, patient's paraphilias may evolve over time in intensity, frequency, and area of desire [8]. Patients who engage in these behaviors may go on to re-offend and may escalate into more serious sexually offensive behaviors, including hands-on offenses. This emphasizes the importance of getting a full chronological history. It is likewise crucial to maintain a sense of nonjudgmental inquiry as the therapeutic alliance continues over time, so that any broadening of the patient's paraphilic repertoire is discovered and addressed in a timely and appropriate manner.

One approach in the assessment of sexual disorders is the four perspectives model—which includes disease, dimension, behavior, and life story. Each individual perspective contributes a distinct feature in formulating a comprehensive case, which still allows for being open to further information and, if necessary, further revision. The disease perspective focuses on the differential diagnosis, and categorizing the disease state, the goal of which is alleviation or cure. The dimension perspective is a measure of an individual's function, and focuses on an individual's relative assets and susceptibilities. This tactic highlights relative strengths, as well as develops strategies to avoid weaknesses. The behavior perspective is focused on goal-directed conduct. With problematic behavior, the objective of the behavior perspective is to interrupt or replace such actions. The fourth and final perspective, the life story perspective, is dependent upon the narrative from the patient, in order to give meaning and perspective to his or her life course. This perspective is utilized when one's life path appears to be taking a destructive turn, with treatment focused on reframing and reconstruction of a life narrative. This perspective is what many associate with psychotherapy, and employs a developmental focus [11].

Once a discussion of actual paraphilic activities has commenced, the clinician must ascertain the level of danger or risk related to the paraphilic behaviors. There may or may not be an immediate danger related to the behavior—for example, as in autoerotic asphyxiation and in some cases of sexual sadism or masochism. In sadism and masochism, the thrill associated with power differential and potential danger is often central to both the masochist's and the sadist's experience [12]. The danger may be benign and symbolic, but could be potentially lethal in actuality. In extreme cases of sadomasochism, where there is loss of control or confusion regarding the boundary between consent and coercion, behaviors can cause physical harm. It is the clinician's task to accurately decipher what is occurring in the sexual experience, on both overt and covert levels. What appears insignificant may hold key details of subtle sexual, intrapsychic, and relational processes that comprise sadomasochistic interactions, which have gone awry. Only a detailed deconstruction of the partners' moment-to-moment interactions permits meaningful decoding of complex sadomasochistic experiences. Evaluation of danger applies to the other paraphilias as well. Once imminent risk has been explored and addressed if necessary, goals of treatment and various treatment modalities can be discussed.

Assessment Tools

While there are various subjective psychometric scales for patient assessment of sexual behaviors [8, 10], clinicians may or may not elect to use these during clinical evaluations. Objective tools and/or structured diagnostic scales also can be utilized in the evaluation of paraphilic patients. The most common objective tools are penile plethysmography, polygraphy, and viewing time of visual stimuli [9, 10]. These techniques have been most widely used in research and with sex offender populations, so their generalizability is unknown.

Penile plethysmography, also called "phallometry," involves measuring the patient's penile response to sexually stimulating material (audiotapes, still photos or slides, or videotapes). Stimuli may vary in content by age and by coercive vs. noncoercive content. Measurements are either taken of changes in penile circumference or changes in penile volume during stimulus presentation. Changes in circumference are recorded via a mechanical device, which the patient himself places on his penis. Changes in penile volume are more complicated, and are measured with the assistance of a technician who helps the patient with proper device placement [10]. Studies using phallometry have been done in male patients with pedophilia, biastophilia, and sexual sadism [13, 14].

Viewing time measurements attempt to draw conclusions between viewing time and specific areas of sexual interests [9, 10, 15]. The Abel Assessment for Sexual Interest (AASI) is a version of viewing time assessments [9, 15]. This combines a self-report survey with measurements of visual reaction times to non-pornographic pictures of people of various ages. Validated assessment instruments have been reviewed including the interrater reliability of the DSM-IV, implicit association task (IAT), viewing time measure and picture association task, which evaluates pedophiles or child sexual abusers [16].

Self-report psychometric tools include the Multidimensional Inventory of Development, Sex and Aggressive behavior (MIDSA), the Multiphasic Sex Inventory (MSI), the Bradford Sexual History Inventory, and the Clarke Sex History Questionnaire for Males-Revised. The MSI is able to distinguish between the types of sexual offenders. The MIDSA, MSI, and SHQ-R assess sexual interests and behaviors [17]. The MIDSA is the most comprehensive as it also covers criminal behavior [14].

The Screening Scale for Pedophilic interests or SSPPI is a four item scale that assesses pedophilic interests such as male victims, more than one child victim, having a victim whose age is 11 years old or younger and having an unrelated child victim among convicted pedophiles and predicts sexual recidivism [14, 18]. The Child Pornography offender risk tool (CPORT) predicts recidivism among adult male sex offenders using child pornography [19].

Affinity 2.5 is a computerized assessment tool, which is based on explicit sexual attractiveness ratings of pictures from both genders combined with viewing time task, which found that pedophilic sexual offenders had higher ratings on attractiveness related to pictures showing small juveniles in explicit rating, as well as in viewing time measures [20]. Visual reaction time measures sexual interest based on how long the individual look at images that are sexually attractive to them. Studies have shown increased visual reaction time can predict recidivism among child sexual offenders [21]. Hempel found that implicit association tasks (IAT) could significantly distinguish between child sexual abusers and non-offenders [22].

Assessment Tools

Objective tools
- Penile plethysmography (phallometry)
- Polygraph
- Viewing Time of Visual Stimuli
  - Abel Assessment for Sexual Interest (AASI)
  - Implicit Association Task (IAT)

Self-report
- Multi-dimensional Inventory of Development, Sex, and Aggressive Behavior (MIDSA)
- Multiphasic Sex Inventory (MSI)
- Bradford Sexual History Inventory
- Clarke Sex History Questionnaire for Males—Revised (SHQ-R)

Screening scales
- Screening Scale for Pedophilic Interests (SSPPI)
- Child Pornography Offender Risk Tool (CPORT)

Computerized assessment tool
- Affinity 2.5

Laboratory Examination

Laboratory examination for paraphilias should incorporate a sexual hormone panel that includes free testosterone, estradiol, progesterone, follicle stimulating hormone (FSH), and luteinizing hormones (LH). Hormone levels are used to establish a baseline level and to screen for abnormal hormonal levels. It also helps to monitor the pharmacological interventions as the hormonal treatment of paraphilias goal is to reduce androgens like testosterone which influences sexual behavior and aggression. Some of these hormones might be helpful in predicting re-offense [14, 23].

Conclusions

In summary, the classification of paraphilia in DSM-IV TR refers to a group of conditions beyond usual love or attraction. As a group, the DSM 5 differentiates between paraphilias and paraphilic disorders, with the major distinction being the level of distress or impairment associated with level of functioning. The evaluation process for paraphilias entails a comprehensive approach, comprised of a psychiatric interview, a longitudinal history, which includes a thorough sexual history. Additionally, collateral information, screening tests, questionnaires, and self-report are useful in assessment. There are various means of assessment utilized in the evaluation of paraphilic disorders, including objective tools, self-reports, screens, and computerized assessment tools. During the evaluation process, it is imperative to consider level of risk associated with paraphilic behaviors, while determining treatment goals.

Case 1: Denial of Erotic Arousal in a Man with Gender Dysphoria

A 37-year-old married man, father of two, sought treatment at a gender identity program with the chief complaint that he wished to become a woman. He reported that he had always felt like a woman but now wanted to transition to that role. He initially denied any fetishistic cross-dressing. His history revealed that he was an outstanding athlete and played football in high school before joining the Marines where he fought in the Middle East and rose to rank of sergeant. Married to his high school sweetheart he has two children. He also reported various extramarital affairs during his marriage but strongly disavowed any same sex interests or behaviors. He continued to masturbate fantasizing himself as a woman. Further history revealed that he recently had lost his business which he started after being discharged from the Marines and was facing serious trouble. After two visits he admitted that his cross-dressing was usually accompanied by extreme fetishistic arousal. Mental status examination revealed a major depressive disorder as well as his gender dysphoria and history of fetishistic cross-dressing. Treatment consisted of active antidepressant pharmacological treatment and supportive psychotherapy.

Comment: This patient initially presented with gender dysphoria and the wish to transition to phenotypic female identity. More extensive evaluation found that the patient was a fetishistic cross dresser despite initial denial of any erotic arousal from wearing feminine clothes. Furthermore, his comorbid depressive diagnosis demanded treatment. The patient eventually chose to disavow his wish for gender transition and remain with his wife as a male. He continued to erotically cross dress in private.

Case 2: A Urinary Issue or Diaper Fetish?

A 29-year-old police officer was seen in psychotherapy for depression. After a few sessions he reported that he required wearing adult diapers due to urinary dribbling. On further questioning he admitted to erotic arousal when he wore such undergarments. The history then emerged that he had always fantasized being an infant and having his diapers changed by his mother. This reverie produced erotic arousal and he would masturbate to the fantasy. The therapy was directed towards the origins of such a preferred arousal pattern. Although the determinants of the paraphilic interest and behavior seemed to reside in his relationship with a distant mother his behavior continued despite enhanced understanding.

Comment: His initial reports of urinary tract issues were at best a rationalization to continue his fetish. Clinicians must be aware of such unusual complaints as a possible sign of a fetish.

References

1. American Psychiatric Association. Diagnostic and statistical manual of mental disorders. 4th ed. Washington, DC: American Psychiatric Association; 2000. p. 553–7.
2. American Psychiatric Association. Diagnostic and statistical manual of mental disorders. 5th ed. Arlington: American Psychiatric Association; 2013.
3. First MB. DSM-5 and paraphilic disorders. J Am Acad Psychiatry Law. 2014;42(2):191–201.

4. Fedoroff JP, Di Gioacchino L, Murphy L. Problems with paraphilias in the DSM-5. Curr Psychiatry Rep. 2013;15(8):363.
5. First MB. DSM-5 proposals for paraphilias: suggestions for reducing false positives related to use of behavioral manifestations. Arch Sex Behav. 2010;39(6):1239–44; author reply 1245–52.
6. Dunsieth Jr NW, Nelson EB, Brusman-Lovins LA, et al. Psychiatric and legal features of 113 men convicted of sexual offenses. J Clin Psychiatry. 2004;65(3):293–300.
7. Gellerman DM, Suddath R. Violent fantasy, dangerousness, and the duty to warn and protect. J Am Acad Psychiatry Law. 2005;33(4):484–95.
8. Firestone P, Kingston DA, Wexler A, Bradford JM. Long-term follow-up of exhibitionists: psychological, phallometric, and offense characteristics. J Am Acad Psychiatry Law. 2006;34(3):349–59.
9. Hall RC, Hall RC. A profile of pedophilia: definition, characteristics of offenders, recidivism, treatment outcomes, and forensic issues. Mayo Clin Proc. 2007;82(4):457–71.
10. Krueger RB, Kaplan MS. Behavioral and psychopharmacological treatment of the paraphilic and hypersexual disorders. J Psychiatr Pract. 2002;8(1):21–32.
11. Fagan PJ. Sexual disorders: perspectives on diagnosis and treatment. Baltimore: Johns Hopkins University Press; 2004.
12. Osborn C, Wise TN. Handbook of sexual dysfunction. Taylor & Francis: Boca Raton; 2005.
13. Seto MC, Ahmed AG. Treatment and management of child pornography use. Psychiatr Clin North Am. 2014;37(2):207–14.
14. Seto MC, Kingston DA, Bourget D. Assessment of the paraphilias. Psychiatr Clin North Am. 2014;37(2):149–61.
15. Lehne G, Thomas K, Berlin F. Treatment of sexual paraphilias: a review of the 1999–2000 literature. Curr Opin Psychiatry. 2000;13(6):569–73.
16. Turner D, Schottle D, Bradford J, Briken P. Assessement methods and management of hypersexuality and paraphilic disorders. Curr Opin Psychiatry. 2014;27(6):413–22.
17. Kingston DA, Seto MC, Firestone P, Bradford JM. Comparing indicators of sexual sadism as predictors of recidivism among adult male sexual offenders. J Consult Clin Psychol. 2010;78(4):574–84.
18. Helmus L, O Ciardha C, Seto MC. The screening scale for pedophilic interests (SSPI): construct, predictive, and incremental validity. Law Hum Behav. 2015;39(1):35–43.

19. Seto MC, Eke AW. Predicting recidivism among adult male child pornography offenders: development of the child pornography offender risk tool (CPORT). Law Hum Behav. 2015;39(4):416–29.
20. Mokros A, Gebhard M, Heinz V. Computarized assessment of pedophilic sexual interest through self report and viewing time; realiability, validity, and classification accuracy of the affinity program. Sex Abuse. 2013;25(3):230–58.
21. Gray SR, Abel GG, Jordan A, Garby T, Wiegel M, Harlow N. Visual reaction time as a predictor of sexual offense recidivism. Sex Abuse. 2015;27(2):173–88.
22. Hempel I, Buck N, Goethals K, van Marle H. Unraveling sexual associations in contact and noncontact child sex offenders using the single category implicit-association test. Sex Abuse. 2013;25(5):444–60.
23. Garcia FD, Delavenne HG, Assumpcao Ade F, Thibaut F. Pharmacologic treatment of sex offenders with paraphilic disorder. Curr Psychiatry Rep. 2013;15(5):356.

Chapter 4
Treatment of Paraphilic Disorders

Deyadira Baez-Sierra, Chandrika Balgobin, and Thomas N. Wise

Treatment of Paraphilias

Overview

As in any therapeutic population, individual paraphilic patients may vary widely in their personal goals of therapy and in which treatment modalities they wish to consider.

Portion of this chapter are modified parts of a chapter previously published in a chapter of Clinical Manual of Sexual Disorders edited by Richard Balon, Robert Taylor Segraves, Chapter: Paraphilic Disorders, Authors: Jeanne M. Lackamp, M.D., Cynthia Osborne, MSW, Thomas N. Wise, M.D., pages 335–370. It has been revised to reflect new data.

D. Baez-Sierra, M.D.
Department of Psychiatry and Behavioral Sciences, George Washington University School of Medicine, Virginia Commonwealth University, Inova Fairfax Hospital, 3300 Gallows Road, Falls Church, VA 22042, USA

Department of Psychiatry, Inova Fairfax Hospital, 3300 Gallows Road, Falls Church, VA 22042, USA

C. Balgobin, D.O.
Department of Psychiatry and Behavioral Sciences, George Washington University School of Medicine, Virginia Commonwealth University, Inova Fairfax Hospital, 3300 Gallows Road, Falls Church, VA 22042, USA

R. Balon (ed.), *Practical Guide to Paraphilia and Paraphilic Disorders*, DOI 10.1007/978-3-319-42650-1_4

Modalities typically include various forms of psychotherapy and/or medication therapy. Along with serotonin reuptake inhibitor antidepressants, other psychiatric medications and androgen deprivation therapy will be reviewed as we describe management and treatment options in both non-coercive and coercive paraphilic patients. The reader will note that emphasis will be placed on the two diagnostic categories about which there has been the most research and writing: transvestic fetishism and pedophilia. These two paraphilias make up the majority of the apprehended sexual offenders.

In 2001, Bradford published an algorithm for the treatment of paraphilias. This algorithm was based on the paraphilias as listed in DSMIII-R. Bradford's algorithm classifies paraphilias from the Level 1 thru 6 according to the severity (mild, moderate, severe, and catastrophic). This algorithm proposes a treatment modality according to the severity of symptoms and impairment. Level 1 proposes treatment with cognitive behavioral therapy (CBT) and relapse prevention for the mild cases. It is recommended regardless of the severity that all patients with paraphilias should be treated with therapy. Level 2 establishes treatment with selective serotonin receptor inhibitors (SSRI). Level 3 is to be considered when symptoms fail to improve with SSRIs within the first 4–6 weeks and adding low dose of medroxyprogesterone (MPA) or cyproterone acetate (CPA) is recommended. Level 4 includes treatment with full dose of oral antiandrogen therapy. Level 5 is designated for severe and catastrophic cases in which long-acting intramuscular hormonal treatment is advised. Level 6 is characterized by the catastrophic

T.N. Wise, M.D. (✉)
Department of Psychiatry, Inova Fairfax Hospital,
3300 Gallows Road, Falls Church, VA 22042, USA

Department of Psychiatry, Johns Hopkins University, Virginia Commonwealth University, George Washington University,
3300 Gallows Road, Falls Church, VA 22042, USA
e-mail: Thomas.Wise@inova.org

paraphilias in which patient failed treatment mentioned above and requires complete androgen suppression with either a higher dose of IM and/or adding additional hormones like luteinizing hormone release hormone (LHRH) [1]. Interestingly, a very similar algorithm was published by Thibaut et al. in 2010. For example Thibaut recommends treatment with gonadotropin release hormone (GnRH) agonists for Level 5 and Level 6 [2].

While psychodynamic psychotherapy has been reported as an intervention for various fetishistic behaviors and transvestism, there is limited evidence for its efficacy [3]. Unfortunately, diagnostic categorization in such case reports often is imprecise, and there are limited outcome measurements verified by external or corroborative methods such as penile plethysmography [4]. This criticism can be made for most treatment interventions in paraphilic patients. Psychodynamic interventions can help the patient better understand issues in his development that led to his present situation, and can potentially allow understanding of the conflicts that fostered paraphilic symptoms [5, 6]. The validity of such conclusions is dependent upon the theoretical stance of the therapist [7]. For instance, does the patient fear women due to castration anxiety or separation from maternal figures, as is found in Freudian theory that has evolved over the decades? [8, 9]. Does the patient have issues that Jungian analytic psychology can illuminate? [10]. Such theoretical approaches may help the therapist organize the data, which the patient presents, but formal psychodynamic outcome studies are lacking in this patient population [11]. The following discussion does not discount psychodynamic methods, but presents the most empirically based data.

General Education

Reviewing the treatment of paraphilias without addressing the basics of patient and family education would be an unfortunate omission. Patient and family should be informed about local law and, e.g., about the painful discrepancy between the legal and psychiatric definition of sexual offenders (the age of the offender and the age difference). Whether or not a patient has presented voluntarily for treatment—unlikely in many cases, due to the ego-syntonic nature of most paraphilias—education of the patient and spouse/family members, and debunking myths of either party, can be helpful in the initial phase of treatment. For instance, one of the most common presentations of transvestic fetishism is that of a patient whom a spouse, partner, or family member has discovered. In these cases, it is essential to understand the other (non-paraphilic) party's perception of the behavior, so that correction of misperceptions and education of the spouse can take place [12]. A spouse may report that she entered the relationship with knowledge of the behavior, while naively assuming that her partner would no longer feel the need to engage in it once in a sexually satisfying marriage. Another may report that she had no knowledge of the behavior until years later when her partner's carelessness led to her accidental discovery; she may even misread the behavior as implying homosexuality. Yet another spouse may report that she knew of the behavior and found it painfully intolerable, but coped with those feelings by a mutual unspoken agreement to ignore it and avoid discussing it. She may have wrongly assumed that she could assume such a stance for the long term, while simultaneously maintaining satisfying emotional and sexual intimacy. These are only some of the common misperceptions family members or spouses may have when attempting to understand their loved one's apparently aberrant sexual behaviors. Education can be beneficial for all involved [12, 13].

It is important to note social skills training, sex education, and even vocational rehabilitation as other possible modalities [13–15]. These all have educational components inherent to them, and are potentially valuable additions to the educational and therapeutic process for paraphilic patients, or patients with paraphilic-type behaviors.

Therapeutic Strategies

The goals for treating the fetishistic cross-dresser will vary depending upon the problems that brought him to seek help. For example, a transvestite who has cross-dressed in secret until his spouse discovers such a behavior may have different treatment aims than the gender dysphoric transvestite who is seeking hormonal therapy. The adolescent whose parents discover his cross-dressing apparel may require counselling to explore how to control such behaviors and keep them private. When the patient verbalizes inability to control his fetishistic activity, antiandrogen treatment could be considered. Finally, it is essential to manage comorbid depression and anxiety both biologically and psychodymically. Treatment data available to date comes from small case reports, open label trials, crossover studies, retrospective studies, meta-analyses, expert consensus, with small sample sizes, lack of control samples, thus the quality of evidence is poor [2, 16]. There is little or no information available to date about the best effective treatment, combination, treatment duration, or the type of offenders. Several review articles suggest the combination of close supervision, pharmacological and behavioral treatment appears to reduce the risk of recidivism.

Treatment of paraphilic disorders raises a plethora of ethical dilemmas since it takes into consideration the balance between public safety, the inclination towards punishment versus treatment, individuals being coerced to treatment by the courts or pressure from others. The treatment guidelines recommendations for the use of hormonal treatment follows the Belgian advisory Committee on Bioethics which hormonal treatment for paraphilic disorders is recommended if the diagnosis of a paraphilic disorder is established by a psychiatrist, there are no contraindications for treatment, the treatment is necessary to prevent serious harm to others or self, no less intrusive means of providing care is available, informed consent for treatment is obtained including informing patient risk versus benefits and treatment plan is in writing that can be modified if necessary [17].

Non-pharmacological Treatments

Cognitive-Behavioral Therapy

Cognitive-behavioral therapy (CBT) is considered the mainstay of treatment in paraphilic patient populations. This is not only cited in numerous papers on paraphilias, but is also reported by the Safer-Society Program and the Association for the Treatment of Sexual Abusers as a widely accepted and effective treatment modality [14, 18, 19]. Just as with pharmacotherapeutic treatments, the majority of literature on CBT in paraphilias focuses on sexual offender populations. The applicability of this may be questionable in the case of a paraphilic patient who has not committed sexual offenses, and this also may be problematic in the case of an individual who has committed a sexual offense but may not suffer from a paraphilia [20]. The merging of cognitive and behavioral approaches is demonstrated below.

Literature on sex offenders indicates that the use of CBT modalities reduces recidivism [20, 21]. There are many aspects to cognitive therapy, some of which include identifying and challenging cognitive distortions, and breaking through patients' denial [14, 21, 22]. *Thought substitution*, *redirection*, and *distractions* are taught as ways to replace maladaptive thoughts and redirect thinking toward more healthy topics. This "cognitive restructuring" is pivotal, as patients learn to challenge and eliminate maladaptive rationalizations, which they use to justify their harmful behaviors [15]. Advanced features of cognitive therapy include *victim empathy training*, which is particularly important in patients with coercive paraphilias [14, 22]. Studer and Aylwin remind us that creating and maintaining rapport in the therapeutic relationship during the course of CBT is as important in the paraphilic population as in any psychiatric patient population [21].

Behavioral methods specific to paraphilias where patients want to focus on decreasing aberrant sexual urges may include *satiation*, *covert sensitization*, *fading*, and *aversive stimulation*. These involve changing the patient's behavioral response to previously sexually exciting stimuli by overuse of the stimuli until response ceases; sensitizing the patient to the stimuli by associating negative outcomes with the stimulus; teaching the patient to mentally transition from aberrant stimuli to more normative stimuli; and making the stimuli frankly unappealing by pairing it with an unpleasant stimulus [14, 18]. Others include *behavioral rehearsal*, *behavioral abstinence*, and *positive conditioning* [23]. These techniques help patients enhance behavioral control along with cognitive control, so that patients can resist urges and make cognitively active choices, instead of automatically thinking and responding in habitual and harmful ways.

Relapse Prevention

Relapse prevention modalities are better known from the field of substance abuse treatment [23, 24]. However, since paraphilias share some features with addictive disorders, some researchers note the utility of relapse prevention in this patient population. Similar to substance abusers, paraphilic patients must learn to navigate a world in which the subject of their preoccupation (whether people of specific ages, particular circumstances, or inanimate objects) is all around them. Identifying risks, learning to deal with urges, and developing a plan of action if faced with a trigger are imperative in this patient population [14, 24]. Research literature in RP proved that does not have an effect in reducing recidivism in a large sample of treated sex offenders. Despite that, RP has become an adjunctive treatment [18, 19].

Motivational Interviewing (MI), Good Lives Model (GLM), and Risk Assessment Model

MI uses an an empathic as well as active approach with the purpose of incentives the individual a commitment for treatment. Good Lives Matter Model is part of the "positive psychology" movement which is based on skills building by enhancing the positive qualities and reaching life fulfilling goals. The Risk Assessment Model approach identifies dynamic risk factors that could be modifiable (versus focusing on past behavior as a predictor of re-offense which cannot be modified). These factors include disregards for others, beliefs that encourages violence towards women or sexual offending, insecure attachments, lack of intimacy, emotional loneliness, poor self-regulation, sexual preoccupation, aberrant sexual interests, and emotional consonance with children. Unfortunately, the risk assessment model does have little or no data supporting the efficacy of this treatment approach [19].

Surgical Castration

Surgical castration used to be the treatment of choice in Europe since the 1800s and in the USA since the 1900s. Surgical castration via bilateral orchiectomy for sex offenders is no longer used in Europe, but is still available in Germany, and in certain states of United States [25]. This option is also available in the Czech Republic with patient consent [26]. According to expert opinion, surgical castration has shown not only reduction in sex re-offense but also a decrease in sexual fantasies. Surgical castration depletes testosterone levels. A side effect of this approach is bone demineralization. One-third of the surgically castrated sexual offenders still engage in sexual intercourse [25], thus increasing the chances for re-offense. Surgical castration can be reverted by using exogenous testosterone [2].

Pharmacological Treatment

Selective Serotonin Reuptake Inhibitors

As noted in the literature, there are no double-blind, randomized, placebo-controlled trials of SSRIs in paraphilic patients [2, 22, 27], but the off-label use of SSRI in the treatment of paraphilias had become the standard of care. It is thought that SSRIs are helpful in treating paraphilias at least in part because they lower sex drive by increasing serotonin [23]. Their side effects are known to include erectile dysfunction, ejaculatory difficulties, and/or reduced libido. The most commonly studied SSRIs for the treatment of paraphilias are sertraline and fluoxetine. Clinical efficacy has been showed at higher doses [28, 29]. Expert consensus recommends its clinical use in mild paraphilias in adolescents, in cases where OCD, impulse control disorder, and depression are comorbid [2, 29]. The Association from the treatment of sexual abusers practice standards recommends the use of SSRI as one intervention to reduce sexual arousal [2]. It should be noted that, in addition to the popularity of using SSRI medications, the tricyclic compound clomipramine also has been used with some success, and its efficacy also has been attributed to its significant serotonin reuptake inhibition [23].

An open label 3 year study using the psychostimulant methylphenidate as adjunctive treatment to SSRI was associated with a decrease in the paraphilia related disorder total sexual outlet score, and mean time spent per day on these behaviors [25].

Hormonal Treatment

Estrogens are no longer used, despite its efficacy in treating paraphilias, due to risk for breast cancer and thromboembolic events among other side effects.

Testosterone and dihydrotestosterone (DHT) are androgens implicated in sexual and aggressive behavior. Higher levels of testosterone have been found in sexual offenders. Steroidal antiandrogens reduce levels of testosterone via feedback inhibition of the hypothalamic pituitary axis and inhibiting the release of luteinizing hormone (LH). Antiandrogen treatment includes cyproterone acetate (not available in the United States), progestogen, medroxyprogesterone acetate (Depo-Provera), and luteinizing hormone-releasing hormone

(LHRH) or gonadotropin-releasing hormone (GNRH) analogues such as "leuprolide acetate" (Depo-Lupron) or "triptorelin" (Trelstar Depot) [14, 15, 22, 30–32]. These compounds work via reduction in testosterone levels, thereby reducing sexual desire and arousal response, and can be administered either orally or via depot injection [14, 22].

Medroxyprogesterone (MPA)

MPA was the first drug studied in the treatment of paraphilias. Besides the hypothalamic pituitary inhibition, MPA increases the metabolism and clearance of testosterone by activating the testosterone alpha reductase. MPA binds to the testosterone-binding globulin, thus decreasing free testosterone. Oral dosage ranges 100–300 mg were used in case reports, double blind and crossover studies. MPA showed efficacy in reducing sexual drive, deviant sexual behavior, and deviant sexual fantasies after 1–2 months [2, 29]. MPA is no longer used in Europe since benefit/risk did not favor the use of MPA. One serious side effect of MPA is pulmonary embolus.

Cyproterone Acetate (CPA)

CPA is a synthetic steroid that binds to androgen brain receptors and acts as a competitive inhibitor of testosterone and DHT. CPA inhibits the release of gonadotropin-releasing hormone (GnRH) and LH. CPA can be given intramuscularly as depot 200–400 mg weekly or every 2 weeks or orally 50–200 mg daily. CPA is mostly used in Middle East, Canada, and Europe. In the USA it is only available in a low dosage form in combination with ethinyl-estradiol. CPA demonstrated efficacy during 4–12 weeks by reducing sexual fantasies and activity in 80–90 % of participants in various studies [2, 28]. Many of the re-offenses have occurred due to non-compliance with treatment.

Gonadotropin-Releasing Hormone Analogs (GnRHa)

GnRH downregulates the secretion of LH and FSH by binding to the pituitary receptors. During the first week of treatment, it can induce an increase in paraphilic sexual behavior due to the LH release and the initial testosterone surge. Cyproterone and flutamide have been used for the testosterone surge. Chronic use of GnRHa causes rapid desensitization of the GnRH receptor, resulting in a decrease of LH. The GnRHa analogs available include triptorelin, leuprorelin, and goserelin. These analogs available in injectable form can be administrated every month with the exception of triptorelin that is also available in a 3 month formulation. There are no studies comparing these three compounds [2, 28, 29]. A 2012 pilot done in a multicenter forensic psychiatric hospital based in Germany double blind controlled clinical trial suggests that the combination of triptorelin and therapy decreased deviant sexual fantasies, urges, and behaviors in paraphilic patients [33]. The duration of treatment with GnRHa remains open. Treatment guidelines suggest a minimal duration treatment of 3–5 years for severe paraphilia with high risk of sexual violence [2, 16]. Efficacy has been maintained as long as the compliance with the antiandrogen continues. The maximal follow-up use was 7–10 years [28].

Because homornal treatments (anti-androgens) foster hypoadrogenism,they include are related to hypoandrogenism which includes, gynecomastia, feminization, asthenia, hot flashes, decreased facial and body hair growth, decreased testicular volume, weight gain, nausea, changes in blood pressure, decreased glucose tolerance, episodic painful ejaculation, diffuse muscular tenderness, sweating, depressive symptoms, bone demineralization, and pain at site of the injection [2, 14, 16, 22, 29–31]. Bone demineralization can be treated with calcium and vitamin d supplementation. Biphosphonates have been effective treating osteopenia and osteoporosis in patients receiving antiandrogens [14]. Contraindications for antiandrogen use includes non-consent, thromboembolic disorder, incomplete puberty, pregnancy, breast feeding, severe hypertension, cardiac and renal diseases, liver failures, severe depression, severe osteoporosis with bone fracture allergy to GnrHa, and active pituitary disease [2, 25]. Of note, some research has found that supplemental "add back" therapy, wherein small doses of testosterone are given back to the patient, can remedy osteoporosis and erectile dysfunction without reactivating paraphilic thoughts [30].

Treatment guidelines recommend to obtain weight, blood pressure, electrocardiogram, bone mineral density, cell blood count, liver functions tests, fasting blood glucose, kidney function test, FSH, LH, testosterone, and prolactin plasma levels prior to initiation of treatment. Depressive symptoms must be evaluated every 1–3 months. Liver enzymes monitoring is required every month for 3 months and then every 3–6 months. Prolactin, glucose, weight, blood cell count, calcium, and phosphate level must be monitored every 6 months and bone mineral density every year. Testosterone levels can be monitored in case of risk of break in therapy or risk of masked testosterone supplementation [2]. Thibaut proposed an algorithm of pharmacological treatment of paraphilias, based on a patient's past medical history, treatment response and compliance, risk of sexual violence, and intensity of paraphilic sexual fantasies. The algorithm uses classification Level 1 through Level 6. Level 1 recommends cognitive behavioral therapy for those paraphilic patients with low risk for sexual violence. Level 2 recommends treatment with high doses of SSRIs for mild paraphilic cases or those who did not respond to CBT alone. Level 3 through Level 6 recommends hormonal treatment. Thibaut recommends all paraphilic patients should be treated with psychotherapy [2].

Other Medications

In addition to antidepressant medications and hormonal medications, other medications may be helpful in some paraphilic patients. Anti-epileptic medications (for instance, topiramate) may be beneficial in treatment of paraphilias such as fetishism [34], as well as other non-paraphilic sexual addiction or compulsions [35, 36]. The hypothesized mechanism of action involves blockage of voltage-gated ion channels, potentiation of GABA (an inhibitory neurotransmitter), and blockage of kainite/AMPA glutamate (excitatory) receptors.

In an interesting case report, Rubenstein and Engel report using lithium and a serotonin reuptake inhibitor in combination to treat a patient's transvestic fetishism, after failure of antidepressant therapies alone [37]. This patient also had tried other medications, including anxiolytics and an antipsychotic. He was not diagnosed with bipolar disorder; rather, lithium was used to augment the antidepressant effect. Not only was the combination of lithium and an SSRI effective in eliminating the patient's behaviors, but he did not suffer orgasmic dysfunction as he had with unopposed antidepressant medications. The authors posited that lithium acted as an "anti-paraphilic augmenter" to the serotonin reuptake inhibitor because of presynaptic serotonin system enhancement [37], again highlighting the importance of serotonin in the manifestation of paraphilias.

Sympathomimetic medications have been cited as helpful for paraphilic patients (or those with paraphilia-related behaviors) who have comorbid attention-deficit hyperactivity disorder [37, 38]. Another study reported that naltrexone, an opiate antagonist, was helpful in a group of adolescent sex offenders. Effectiveness was measured by reduction in frequency of sexual fantasies and masturbatory activity [39]. Federoff published a case of transvestic fetishism treated successfully with buspirone [40]. Treatment with dopamine blockers including chlorpromazine, benperidol, and fluphenazine have been mentioned in the literature with mixed results [2].

Finally, Varela and Black reported successful treatment of a pedophilic patient with a combination of carbamazepine and clonazepam [41]. The patient had significant anxiety and dysphoria associated with his pedophilic behaviors, but otherwise had no comorbid psychiatric diagnoses. Once started on the medications above, his unwanted thoughts and behaviors ceased, and his success was noted to have lasted 1 year (at time of case report publication).

Although the above reports focus on individual patients or small groups of patients, they serve as evidence that these challenging psychiatric disorders may require therapeutic and pharmacologic creativity on the part of treating clinicians. Admittedly, more research needs to be done, but the potential for successful treatment using these and other medications should be noted and pursued.

Case 1

A 45-year-old attorney was evaluated with his wife who complained that she was "sick and tired" of his cross-dressing. He replied that this was his favorite activity.

The patient reported that he began dressing when he was 13 after trying on his mother's underwear and found this intensely exciting. He would fantasize during masturbation that he was wearing feminine clothes while having intercourse with woman. At no point did he admit to same sex fantasies or experience. He regularly used female underwear that he bought via mail order during his adolescence but stopped such behaviors during college since he didn't want to be discovered by his roommates. He felt his parents had no idea of his fetishistic behavior. During law school his cross-dressing reemerged and he correlated this to anxiety about his classes. He began dating his wife and eventually told her about his behavior. She reported that she believed after marriage he would stop cross-dressing. He would increasingly ask her if he could wear a feminine nightgown to bed but she refused and he became irritable. After the couple had two children she began to fear they would discover his behavior and sought psychiatric evaluation. The patient presented as heterosexually oriented. He admitted to a few affairs with coworkers on business trips and had basically masculine interests such as hunting. He said that when he cross-dressed he was expressing another part of his personality. He never cross-dressed in public but privately collected pornography of cross-dressed men having intercourse with woman. Each member of the couple entered individual psychotherapy. He was able to better understand that anxiety increased his wish to cross-dress and he reported less anxiety with antidepressants and was able to greatly reduce his fetishistic activity but still was excited by erotic fantasies of himself cross-dressed. He was not interested in gender reassignment or was gender dysphoric. His wife was displeased with his behavior but decided in therapy that the other parts of the marriage were sufficient to continue in the relationship. "He is basically a good man."

Discussion: This typifies a clinical situation wherein a couple presents with the man endorsing enjoyable fetishistic cross-dressing. Individual therapy is the best approach to let each member of the dyad understand their behavior and the pros and cons of remaining in the relationship. Couples therapy is complex since the transvestite cannot easily "stop" cross-dressing nor is it easy for many woman to leave the marriage. Thus in treating the fetishistic cross-dresser the first goal is to ascertain whether depression and/or anxiety are increasing the drive to cross-dress and examine the elements of such affective distress. The therapy should review the life story of each patient to try to understand the individual. One goal in such cases is for the cross-dresser to understand the effect of this behavior upon their partner and thus try to better limit cross-dressing or at least practice such fetishistic acts privately.

Case 2

A 56-year-old government employee presented for a psychiatric evaluation due to a long-standing behavior of being sexually aroused by wearing diapers. He initially noted he did this due to urinary dribbling but upon closer questioning he admitted that he ejaculated when wearing such undergarments. He sought the evaluation when his wife who had become a chronic alcoholic was so angry and demeaning to him about his diaper fetish. He reported that he began to wear such objects in his later adolescents although he fantasized about this during masturbatory activity beginning a few years before actually trying the diapers. His fantasies involved his being a young child who is being spanked by his mother. His childhood history revealed an abusive mother who was an alcoholic. His father a passive man enabled her and never stopped his wife from verbal and mild physical abuse of the patient. Therapy was directed towards initially trying to get his wife into substance abuse treatment which he could not. He also began to see that his anxiety was escalated by his wife's behavior which was similar to his mother's outbursts and his fetish has some symbolism about the fantasy that he could finally get his mother to resist such abuse.

Comment: The patient's wife recreated his maternal experience. When this was discussed it offered some insight and mobilized the patient to try to induce his wife into active treatment. His anxiety lessened and he could control his paraphilia better than when he began therapy. As with case 1 the goal is to first treat the affective disorder if present but also try to get the patient to understand the course of his paraphilia—when it began, when it escalates, and how it effects others. It is often impossible to stop such behaviors in preferred erotic fantasies or in practice.

Case 3

A 40-year-old married father of a 12-year-old son was evaluated in the Emergency Room of a large hospital for hematuria. Evaluation revealed small petechial looking lesions on his scrotum which he admitted to being pinprick in that he would put pins into his scrotum and into the testes. He reported excruciating pain but found it so sexually arousing that he would repeatedly do this and would lead to ejaculation. He reported that as a teen he would squeeze his scrotum during masturbation with the resulting pain heightening his erotic pleasure despite the pain. The repertoire escalated to tying his testes with rubber bands and finally to inserting pins into his genitals. He denied any suicidal ideation or behaviors and had no concurrent psychiatric diagnoses. He was referred for a psychiatric evaluation. His first topics during the initial psychiatric visit was his anger at overhearing the Emergency Room staff laughing about his behavior. He described a childhood without trauma. His father was often away due to his work while his mother was a loving although controlling parent. He had a brother whom he described as normal. He dated during adolescence and was popular during his college years. His wife did not know about his masochistic behavior and never observed his scrotum. He would avoid intimacy when he developed orchiditis after such behaviors. His preferred masturbatory fantasies beginning in adolescence were images of a powerful woman with a razor threatening him with castration but never follows through. The therapy attempted to elaborate upon this theme to foster some insight into his attitudes towards female figures and specifically his mother but he would not associate to the behavior just noting "it is what it is." He left therapy after five visits.

Comment: In contradistinction to the above cases, the paraphilic behavior in this patient must be stopped. The patient has to understand how dangerous it is to his health. This is a difficult task but as with all behavioral disorders the triggers that foster the actual paraphilic act should be identified and safer erotic patterns developed. This could include fantasies but not actual dangerous behaviors. It may be difficult for patients to admit continuation of such behaviors to their therapists but ongoing treatment would hopefully develop a working therapeutic alliance with trust and openness.

The family constellation of many paraphilic man suggests that anger towards controlling maternal figures maybe a useful construct but often such patients are unable to utilize such ideas in a constructive manner and could be considered alexithymic in that they have a concrete manner of thinking denoted as an operational style of cognition. The lack of specificity of the triad of a distant father and controlling mother make etiological factors difficult upon which to generalize.

References

1. Bradford JM. The neurobiology, neuropharmacology and pharmacological treatment of paraphilias and compulsive sexual behavior. Can J Psychiatry. 2001;46:26–34.
2. Thibaut F, De La Barra F, Gordon H, Cosyns P, Bradford JM. WFSBP Task Force on Sexual Disorders. The world federation of societies of biological psychiatry (WFSBP) guidelines for the biological treatment of paraphilias. World J Biol Psychiatry. 2010;11(4):604–55.
3. Bemporad JR, Dunton HD, Spady FH. Case reports the treatment of a child foot fetishist. Am J Psychother. 1976;30(2): 303–16.
4. Greenacre P. The transitional object and the fetish with special reference to the role of illusion. Int J Psychoanal. 1970;51(4): 447–56.
5. McHugh PR, Slavney PR. Methods of reasoning in psychopathology: conflict and resolution. Compr Psychiatry. 1982;23(3):197–215.
6. Wise TN. Psychotherapy of an aging transvestite. J Sex Marital Ther. 1979;5(4):368–73.
7. McHugh PR, Slavney PR. Perspectives in psychiatry. 2nd ed. Baltimore: Johns Hopkins University Press; 1998.
8. Bak RC. Distortions of the concept of fetishism. Psychoanal Study Child. 1974;29:191–214.
9. Freud and fetishism: Previously unpublished minutes of the Vienna psychoanalytic society. Psychoanal Q. 1988;57(2):147–66.
10. Springer A. Female perversion: scenes and strategies in analysis and culture. J Anal Psychol. 1996;41(3):325–38.
11. Frank JD, Frank JB. Persuasion and healing: a comparative study of psychotherapy. Baltimore: Johns Hopkins University Press; 1993.
12. Wise TN, Fagan PJ, Schmidt CW, Ponticas Y, Costa PT. Personality and sexual functioning of transvestitic fetishists and other paraphilics. J Nerv Ment Dis. 1991;179(11):694–8.
13. Coleman E, Siributr P, Leelamanit V, Tapanya S. The treatment of fetishism and socially inappropriate sexual behavior in a young male with dull normal intelligence. J Med Assoc Thai. 1993;76(9):531–4.
14. Krueger RB, Kaplan MS. Behavioral and psychopharmacological treatment of the paraphilic and hypersexual disorders. J Psychiatr Pract. 2002;8(1):21–32.

15. Sadock BJ, Sadock VA. Kaplan and Sadock's synopsis of psychiatry: behavioral sciences/clinical psychiatry. Philadelphia: Lippincott Williams & Wilkins; 2011.
16. Garcia FD, Thibaut F. Current concepts in the pharmacotherapy of paraphilias. Drugs. 2011;71(6):771–90.
17. Belgian Advisory Commitee on Bioethics. Opinion no. 39 of december 18th 2006 on hormonal treatment of sex offenders. http://www.health.belgium.be/eportal/Healthcare/Consultativebodies/Commitees/Bioethics/Opinions/index.htm#.VhrEDij_ZFI. Updated 2006. Accessed Oct 11, 2015.
18. Kaplan MS, Krueger RB. Cognitive-behavioral treatment of the paraphilias. Isr J Psychiatry Relat Sci. 2012;49(4):291–6.
19. Marshall WL, Marshall LE. Psychological treatment of the paraphilias: a review and an appraisal of effectiveness. Curr Psychiatry Rep. 2015;17(6):47.
20. Lehne G, Thomas K, Berlin F. Treatment of sexual paraphilias: a review of the 1999–2000 literature. Curr Opin Psychiatry. 2000;13(6):569–73.
21. Studer LH, Aylwin AS. Pedophilia: the problem with diagnosis and limitations of CBT in treatment. Med Hypotheses. 2006;67(4):774–81.
22. Hall RC, Hall RC. A profile of pedophilia: definition, characteristics of offenders, recidivism, treatment outcomes, and forensic issues. Mayo Clin Proc. 2007;82(4):457–71.
23. Osborn C, Wise TN. Handbook of sexual dysfunction. Boca Raton: Taylor & Francis; 2005.
24. Brunette MF, Mueser KT. Psychosocial interventions for the long-term management of patients with severe mental illness and co-occurring substance use disorder. J Clin Psychiatry. 2006;67 Suppl 7:10–7.
25. Guay DR. Drug treatment of paraphilic and nonparaphilic sexual disorders. Clin Ther. 2009;31(1):1–31.
26. Stojanovski V. Surgical castration of sex offenders and its legality: the case of czech republic. http://www.iusetsocietas.cz/fileadmin/user_upload/Vitezne_prace/Stojanovski.pdf. Accessed Nov 30, 2015.
27. Briken P, Kafka MP. Pharmacological treatments for paraphilic patients and sexual offenders. Curr Opin Psychiatry. 2007;20(6):609–13.
28. Garcia FD, Delavenne HG, Assumpcao Ade F, Thibaut F. Pharmacologic treatment of sex offenders with paraphilic disorder. Curr Psychiatry Rep. 2013;15(5):356.

29. Assumpcao AA, Garcia FD, Garcia HD, Bradford JM, Thibaut F. Pharmacologic treatment of paraphilias. Psychiatr Clin North Am. 2014;37(2):173–81.
30. Briken P, Hill A, Berner W. Pharmacotherapy of paraphilias with long-acting agonists of luteinizing hormone-releasing hormone: a systematic review. J Clin Psychiatry. 2003;64(8):890–7.
31. Rosler A, Witztum E. Treatment of men with paraphilia with a long-acting analogue of gonadotropin-releasing hormone. N Engl J Med. 1998;338(7):416–22.
32. Briken P, Hill A, Berner W. A relapse in pedophilic sex offending and subsequent suicide attempt during luteinizing hormone-releasing hormone treatment. J Clin Psychiatry. 2004;65(10):1429.
33. Briken P, Berner W. P278 study group. Double-blind, controlled, clinical trial planned in Germany to investigate the efficacy of psychotherapy combined with triptorelin in adult male patients with severe pedophilic disorders: presentation of the study protocol. Isr J Psychiatry Relat Sci. 2012;49(4):306–13.
34. Shiah IS, Chao CY, Mao WC, Chuang YJ. Treatment of paraphilic sexual disorder: the use of topiramate in fetishism. Int Clin Psychopharmacol. 2006;21(4):241–3.
35. Fong TW, De La Garza 2nd R, Newton TF. A case report of topiramate in the treatment of nonparaphilic sexual addiction. J Clin Psychopharmacol. 2005;25(5):512–4.
36. Khazaal Y, Zullino DF. Topiramate in the treatment of compulsive sexual behavior: case report. BMC Psychiatry. 2006;6:22.
37. Rubenstein EB, Engel NL. Successful treatment of transvestic fetishism with sertraline and lithium. J Clin Psychiatry. 1996;57(2):92.
38. Kafka MP, Hennen J. Psychostimulant augmentation during treatment with selective serotonin reuptake inhibitors in men with paraphilias and paraphilia-related disorders: a case series. J Clin Psychiatry. 2000;61(9):664–70.
39. Ryback RS. Naltrexone in the treatment of adolescent sexual offenders. J Clin Psychiatry. 2004;65(7):982–6.
40. Fedoroff JP. Buspirone hydrochloride in the treatment of transvestic fetishism. J Clin Psychiatry. 1988;49(10):408–9.
41. Varela D, Black DW. Pedophilia treated with carbamazepine and clonazepam. Am J Psychiatry. 2002;159(7):1245–6.

Chapter 5
Voyeuristic Disorder

Richard Balon

Introduction

In psychiatry, sexuology, and sexual medicine, voyeurism/voyeuristic disorder is conceptualized as a condition characterized by deriving intense and recurrent sexual arousal from watching unsuspecting person(s) while they are having sex, disrobe, or are nude. It has been classified as one of the exploitive paraphilias/paraphilic disorders. Acts of voyeurism are probably the most common of potentially law-breaking sexual behaviors [1]. Voyeurism in contemporary psychiatry and sexual medicine terms should not be confused with the popular culture definition of voyeurism. As Metzl [2] pointed out, popular definitions of voyeurism are as broad as psychiatric definitions are narrow. He notes the difference between a "relatively expansive category of acceptable voyeurism"

R. Balon, M.D. (✉)
Department of Psychiatry and Behavioral Neurosciences, Wayne State University, Tolan Park Building, 3rd Floor, 3901 Chrysler Service Dr., Detroit, MI 48201, USA

Department of Anesthesiology, Wayne State University, Tolan Park Building, 3rd Floor, 3901 Chrysler Service Dr., Detroit, MI 48201, USA
e-mail: rbalon@wayne.edu

R. Balon (ed.), *Practical Guide to Paraphilia and Paraphilic Disorders*, DOI 10.1007/978-3-319-42650-1_5

which is a late twentieth-century phenomenon and a narrow category of pathological voyeurism and voyeuristic disorder in the psychiatric sense. Metzl ([2], p 127) further writes that while "contemporary American psychiatry seems to struggle to identify a population of voyeurs who are, in fact, sick enough to require treatment with psychotherapy and psychotropic medication… evidence also suggests that the notion of voyeurism has limited relevance in a world where it is at times difficult to distinguish hard-core paraphiliacs who require psychiatric interventions from the many amateurs who simply watch VTV ("voyeurism TV") programs." The notion of pathological and "normal" voyeurism and the difference between those two terms/entities is very important, as the line between pathology and what our society considers "normal" or acceptable is becoming more blurry.

It seems that many so-called "normal" people have a tendency to be involved in voyeurism in the sense that psychiatry considers paraphilia or paraphilic tendencies. We have no data on how many people watch adult pornography over the Internet or through other technological means, but it seems that the pornography industry is flourishing. Are all those who watch people disrobing or having sex voyeurs? Are we a voyeur nation/culture that just does not want to admit it? Are many of us voyeurs just afraid of being caught or admit it? In an interesting study Rye and Meaney [3] tried to determine whether "normal" people would engage in voyeurism. They asked university students about the likelihood of them secretly watching an attractive person undressing or two attractive people having sex, both being hypothetical situations. The chance of being caught was manipulated (e.g., 0, 10, or 25 %). The participants in this study (aptly called "Voyeurism: it is good as long as we do not get caught") reported a willingness to watch an attractive person undress, provided they would not be caught. Fewer participants (more males than females) reported a willingness to watch a sexual activity under similar circumstances. When the risk of being caught increased, the likelihood of watching decreased (from 84 to 61 % in men, and from 74 to 36 % in women). These findings shed a little bit of light on the question of whether many people have a tendency toward voyeurism. However, these findings also raise questions about the definition (DSM and ICD) of voyeurism/voyeuristic disorder and what Downing [4] calls DSM bias in favor of heteronormativity and reproduction.

Voyeurism has been a known phenomenon since the ancient times. Aggrawal [5] notes several descriptions of voyeurism in the Bible, namely the case of King David who got sexually aroused watching unsuspecting Bathsheba taking a bath. King David's solution to his sexual urges were different than what has been considered as resolution of voyeuristic urges and fantasies in the literature and by the public. King David had sex with Bathsheba, arranged for the "departure" of her husband Uriah and Bathsheba later gave King David a son, Solomon. In the contemporary view, a person suffering from voyeuristic disorder is a "Peeping Tom" watching an unsuspecting person, while probably masturbating.

Interestingly, the literature on voyeurism is relatively scarce. In the first review of the literature on voyeurism Smith [6] wrote that "the most striking thing about the literature on voyeurism is the relative lack of material in print." At that time (1976), Smith [6] found only 15 articles and no books dealing specifically with voyeurism. The situation has not changed much. The two most comprehensive clinically oriented reviews of voyeurism are two chapters [7, 8] in a book on *Sexual deviance* [9] by Laws and O'Donohue from 2008. Thus a lot of guidance on managing voyeurism/voyeuristic disorder is based on scarce evidence and assumptions.

Diagnostic Criteria

The basic diagnostic concept of voyeurism as watching an unsuspecting person either naked, disrobing, or engaged in sexual activity while achieving sexual excitement has been kept across various diagnostic classifications and editions of the Diagnostic and Statistical Manual of Mental Disorders (DSM). Interestingly, the earlier editions of the DSM are clearer on what sexual excitement means. The DSM-III [10] states (p 272) that, "Orgasm, usually produced by masturbation, may occur during the voyeuristic activity, or later, in response to the memory of what the individual has witnessed." The text continues, "Often, these individuals enjoy thinking about the observed individuals' being helpless and feeling humiliated if they knew they were being seen. In its severe form, peeping constitutes the exclusive form of sexual activity" (p 272–273). The DSM-5 [11] does not address the issue of achieving sexual excitement. It deals mostly with the newly created distinction between voyeurism and voyeuristic disorder. The International Classification of Diseases (ICD) definitions are not discussed here as they are fairly limited in earlier editions and the 11th edition is still in the making.

The DSM-5 criteria of voyeuristic disorder ([11], p 686–687) are as follows (Reprinted with permission from the Diagnostic and Statistical Manual of Mental Disorders, Fifth Edition, (Copyright 2013). American Psychiatric Association.):

Criterion A: Over a period of at least 6 months, recurrent and intense sexual arousal from observing an unsuspecting person who is naked, in the process of disrobing, or engaging in sexual activity, as manifested by fantasies, urges or behaviors.

Criterion B: The individual has acted on these sexual urges with a nonconsenting person, or the sexual urges or fantasies cause clinically significant distress or impairment in social, occupational, or other important areas of functioning

Criterion C: The individual experiencing the arousal and/or acting on the urges is at least 18 years of age.

Specify:
In controlled environment: This specifier is primarily applicable to individuals living in institutional or other settings where opportunities to engage in voyeuristic behavior are restricted.
In full remission: The individual has not acted on the urges with a nonconsenting person, and there has been no distress or impairment in social, occupational or other areas of functioning, for at least 5 years while in an uncontrolled environment.

There are several points of the DSM-5 criteria that need some clarification or attention. The first issue is the clear distinction between voyeurism and voyeuristic disorder. To fulfill the criteria for a disorder, the individual has to act on sexual urges with a nonconsenting person. As mentioned before, to act in general understanding of voyeurism means to watch an unsuspecting person and achieve excitement through masturbation and no sexual activity with the person watched is sought. The DSM-5 language is, unfortunately, vague on this issue. The Criterion B statement that "The individual has acted on these sexual urges with a nonconsenting person…" is open to various interpretations. What does it mean acting on sexual urges with a nonconsenting person? Most experts would agree that it means watching/getting excited without consent of the watched person and that "acting" means watching and masturbating, but the DSM-5 terminology is vague. The language is even more confusing in the Diagnostic Features part of the DSM-5 ([11], p 687) where the text states that "Recurrent voyeuristic behavior constitutes sufficient support for voyeurism (by fulfilling Criterion A) and simultaneously demonstrates that this paraphilically motivated behavior is causing harm to others (by fulfilling Criterion B)." The harm to others is not clear if the person is unsuspecting. Confusion is also created by using the word "unsuspecting" in Criterion A and "nonconsenting" in Criterion B.

The second issue is the non-consenting character of the person being watched. As discussed before, many people get excited by watching pornography through various media, or watching a prostitute or a partner disrobing. Again, interestingly, DSM-5 [11] is not as clear on this issue as DSM-III and other DSM editions are. The text of DSM-III states that, "Watching pornography, filmed or live, causes sexual excitement. However, the people who are being observed are willingly in view, even though in fantasy the observer may *imagine* (but knows better) that the people are unsuspecting" ([10], p 273). Thus, the distinction of voyeurism/voyeuristic disorder and voyeuristic behavior/watching pornography has to be carefully parsed during the clinical evaluation.

The third issue is the addition of Criterion C, i.e., that the person experiencing and acting on urges must be at least 18 years old. As DSM-5 points out, puberty and adolescence increase curiosity and activity in various areas, including sexuality, and thus this criterion was added to alleviate the risk of pathologizing normative sexual interest and behavior during this developmental period. Children and adolescents under the age of 18 peeking at people who are naked, disrobing, or having sex should not be necessarily labeled as suffering from voyeurism/voyeuristic disorder.

Summary of Evidence

Voyeuristic acts are frequently called the most common of potentially law-breaking sexual behaviors ([11], p 687), yet we really do not know how frequent voyeurism/voyeuristic disorder is. The highest cited lifetime prevalence is estimated to be 12 % in males and 4 % in females. Like most other paraphilias/paraphilic disorders, voyeurism/voyeuristic behavior is more common among men. The voyeurism/voyeuristic disorder in women is less well understood than in men. Smith [6] in his review concluded that the voyeur is a relatively young man of low socioeconomic status, who "sociosexually is said to be 'not retarded but a late bloomer.' He is prone to minor crimes and not major offenses." However, there is a certain number of voyeurs with a late onset.

The etiology of voyeurism/voyeuristic disorder is unknown. There are various theories attempting to explain the voyeuristic behavior—psychoanalytic, social learning, lovemaps, courtship, sociobiological (evolutionary: men "inspecting" women for the most suitable partner), and biological. However, as with all paraphilias/paraphilic disorders, these are just theories of etiology.

The cornerstone of assessment of a person accused of/suspected of/distressed about voyeuristic acts is a good comprehensive clinical interview. Mann and colleagues [8] suggest that clinical interview should cover the following areas: features of hypersexuality and compulsivity of voyeuristic behavior (could provide a clue for treatment); sexual and emotional intimacy, including attachment patterns; sexual fantasy content; beliefs about the deviance/harm of voyeurism; sexual self-esteem and body image; impact on relationship and body image; anxiety and depression; hostility; and lifestyle and environmental factors (some occupations and hobbies provide opportunities for voyeurism). There are also sexual history questionnaires that include questions about voyeurism, but these are usually long (hundreds of questions), not validated and probably not clinically useful.

Information about treatment of voyeurism is scarce and treatment efficacy is frequently assumed based on preferred theories of etiology of the treating professional, or on effectiveness of treatment in other paraphilias/paraphilic disorders. For instance, early case reports suggested behavioral approach to extinguish voyeuristic behavior. Jackson [12] reported a case in which a male self-referred for peeping into windows for several years without being caught. A survey of potentially exciting stimuli revealed that pornographic pictures had the maximum arousing properties after voyeurism. It was suggested that he masturbates in the privacy of his bedroom to the most exciting pornographic picture he possessed next time he felt an urge to peep. He was told to focus on the picture at the time of orgasm. At the end of 2 weeks of following these instructions he reported no desire to look into windows. The treatment continued for 8 sessions (using pairing of his orgasm with a nude picture). Nine months after termination of his treatment he reported that his desire for voyeurism dissipated.

Mann and colleagues [8] summarized possible treatments of voyeurism/voyeuristic disorder. They pointed out that the goal of treatment should be the reduction of voyeurism, while maintaining the frequency of sexual behavior, either heterosexual or homosexual. They also noted, citing the previous edition of Laws and O'Donohue book [9] that there is not enough solid and consistent evidence in the literature to support or prefer any treatment and that any treatment of voyeurism should be considered experimental. That was written in 2008 and the situation is not different in 2016. As Balon [13] pointed out, it is not clear what exactly should be treated and what the goals of treatment should be. Should the goal be the extinction of urges or fantasies, or should it be the extinction of voyeuristic behavior? Should the distress be a guiding treatment principle? The answer is that distress probably should not be a guiding principle, as society would not consider it to be enough. We do not know much about the course of the disorder—thus the length of treatment is also not clear and should be guided by clinical symptomatology, and may be also be guided by the courts (mandated treatment for sexual offense).

Mann and colleagues ([8], p 327) also noted that "The approach of choice at any given time period reflects the dominant therapeutic tradition of the day: reports of psychoanalytic treatment in the 1950s and 1960s, behavioral therapies in the 1970s and early 1980s, and pharmacological treatments in the 1990s and beyond 2000." The reports on the efficacy are usually just case reports or case series, at best.

There have been several cases of successful treatment of voyeurism with selective serotonin reuptake inhibitors (SSRIs) reported in the literature. Emmanuel, Lydiard, and Ballenger [14] used fluoxetine (up to 60 mg/day) in a patient with ego dystonic voyeurism, which he was unable to resist. They selected fluoxetine based on some similarities of paraphilic behavior and obsessive-compulsive behavior, and they were also inspired by a case of exhibitionism responding to fluoxetine [15]. Abouesh and Clayton [16] described the case of a voyeur whose voyeuristic behavior decreased in frequency as well as in intensity of his urges on 20 mg of paroxetine at bedtime. He discontinued his treatment after 3 months, as he was doing well. He continued to do well in at a 4-months follow-up after treatment discontinuation.

Krueger and Kaplan [17] treated 12 men suffering from different paraphilias with depot leuprolide acetate, a synthetic gonadotropin-releasing hormone receptor agonist. Three of these men were diagnosed with voyeurism (in addition to other paraphilias, one suffered from voyeurism, exhibitionism, and frotteurism, one from voyeurism and pedophilia, and one from voyeurism and exhibitionism; two of them had other psychiatric diagnoses). Subjects received depot-leuprolide acetate 7.5 mg monthly. To counteract a surge of follicle-stimulating hormone and luteinizing hormone (and thus testosterone), they also received flutamide 250 mg three times a day for 30 days. These three subjects were treated for 6, 12, and 35 months, respectively. All three reported decreased sexual arousal and their testosterone level dropped precipitously to a very low level. The side effects of leuprolide acetate were serious, including gynecomastia and decreased bone density.

Treatment of voyeurism/voyeuristic disorder is clearly unchartered territory, similar or even less known than other paraphilias/paraphilic disorders. Most of the recommended approaches are based on case reports or derived from the experience with other paraphilias/paraphilic disorders. In his algorithm for treatment of paraphilias, Bradford [18, 19] recommended that "regardless of the severity of the paraphilia, cognitive-behavioral treatment and relapse-prevention treatment would always be given" ([19], p 29–30). In cases of mild or moderate paraphilias, pharmacological treatment should start with SSRIs. If SSRIs were not effective, Bradford suggests to administer a small dose of antiandrogens (e.g., 50 mg of medroxyprogesterone acetate [MPA] or cyproterone acetate [CPA]), this would be used in mild or moderate levels of paraphilia. The moderate to severe levels of paraphilias would require full oral antiandrogen doses (50–300 mg of MPA or CPA). More serious levels would require intramuscular MPA weekly or CPA every other week. The catastrophic level of paraphilia would require higher doses of intramuscular CPA, a luteinizing hormone-releasing hormone (LHRH). It should be emphasized that psychological and pharmacological approaches should always be combined.

We can probably assume that the treatment of "pure" voyeurism/voyeuristic disorder is not going to reach catastrophic levels suggested by Bradford and thus treatment of "pure" voyeurism/voyeuristic disorder would not need hormonal intervention. Combination of various therapies, self-help, and SSRIs may suffice. However, as paraphilias/paraphilic disorders frequently coexist with another one or overlap like in Krueger and Kaplan [17] cases, more aggressive treatment may be needed in many cases.

Clinical Example (Fictitious Case Made Up/Anonymized from Several Cases)

A 30-year-old man was referred for evaluation after several complaints to his supervisor that he had been observed peeking in the windows at the student dormitory, where he works as a night guard. The students did not report any unusual behavior or attempts to contact them on his part, just that several of them noticed him standing outside at night and looking in their or others' windows. They felt uncomfortable. When approached by one of the students who was returning to the dormitory late and noticed him standing in the shadows, he stated he was making sure "everything was OK and safe."

During the initial part of the examination, he insisted that he had done nothing wrong, "just taking care of security at the dorm." He appeared to be quite anxious and admitted to being "a bit depressed." He denied a history of treatment for depression or any other issues. The patient reported living alone in a small apartment. He had several girlfriends in the past with whom he had a sexual relationship. He said that these relationships were "nothing serious, nothing exciting." He is a loner, likes to play on his computer or watching TV. He admitted getting drunk "a few times a month, the only times I feel better."

He graduated from the high school and attended college for several years. He studied liberal arts and history, never obtained a degree. He added, "I am going to complete my studies one of these days." He has had several jobs, as a security guard and as a clerk. He has been in his present job for 8 months. He reluctantly admitted that he was fired from a previous job for a similar issue, "I was making sure everything was OK and they claimed I was intruding on people's privacy."

He was reluctant to talk about his childhood and adolescence during his initial evaluation. He opened gradually during the subsequent couple of sessions. He admitted that he has been masturbating while watching female students disrobing or getting dressed—"can you imagine, they walk naked there." He was even more excited when "I was occasionally lucky when I saw them having sex… I daydreamed about it at home, masturbating." He was more excited about watching unsuspecting women than by other sex related activities "since I was a kid, about 15, and saw the neighbor's daughter changing her clothes and later having sex with her boyfriend." He did not describe his urges as being intrusive or of obsessive-compulsive character, but rather as a matter of opportunity of being able to watch, or as frustration of not having sex for a long time. He said that sex with his girlfriends was "OK, but not as exciting as watching someone else. I also asked a couple of girls to disrobe in front of me, but the excitement was not the same as when I watched someone who did not know, and these girls did not like that I just masturbated when watching them and that I did not want to have sex afterwards." He was upset about not being able to keep a permanent relationship with any girl, "they all left me, complaining about my performance." He never told anybody about watching unsuspecting women or couples and masturbating. He said he felt relieved that he was finally able to talk to someone about it, as "I don't know what to do…."

After a discussion of the therapeutic options, he was referred for individual therapy (combination of psychoeducation and cognitive behavioral therapy). He was also started on fluoxetine 20 mg/day, the dose was later increased to 40 mg. He reported relief of his depression and anxiety, and a decrease of sexual urges and fantasies later on. He continues in therapy and on fluoxetine 40 mg/day. He reports occasional urges to watch, but has not been acting on them. He masturbates occasionally while watching pornographic movies. He has entertained the idea of "starting to date seriously."

Recommendations

Patients with suspected or confirmed voyeurism/voyeuristic disorder should be carefully evaluated to determine the presence of voyeurism/voyeuristic disorder. A detailed clinical interview should be the cornerstone of the initial evaluation.

The approach to the patient should be nonjudgmental, empathic. The evaluation should focus on urges, fantasies, behaviors, and also on overlap with other paraphilias/paraphilic disorders and on comorbidity with other mental disorders (e.g., personality disorders and substance use disorders). The evaluating clinician should be careful in evaluating young males at the end of puberty, or around the age of 18, to distinguish between true voyeurism/voyeuristic disorder and age-appropriate puberty-related sexual curiosity and activity ([11], p 688). The clinical interview should also focus on issues such as hypersexuality and compulsivity of the voyeuristic behavior, sexual fantasy content, beliefs about deviance/harm to others, self-esteem and body image, impact on relationships and social functioning, anxiety, depression, hostility, lifestyle, and environmental factors [8].

The treatment of voyeurism should start with developing the therapeutic relationship and an atmosphere of trust. Therapy, namely CBT and relapse-prevention, should be the first step in the management of this disorder. Use of self-help books or referrals to programs such as Sexaholics Anonymous me also help. SSRIs such as fluoxetine and paroxetine should be added if there is no improvement. Hormonal therapy should be reserved for cases resistant to SSRIs and psychotherapy, for cases of recidivism and for cases encompassing several paraphilias/paraphilic disorders, especially those causing more harm to others, e.g., sadistic disorder or pedophilic disorder. Combining various treatments seems prudent, though there is no evidence addressing treatment combinations. Treatment risks and side effects should always be discussed with the patient, even in cases of court-mandated treatment.

References

1. Langstrom N. The DSM diagnostic criteria for exhibitionism, voyeurism, and frotteurism. Arch Sex Behav. 2010;39:317–24.
2. Metzl JM. Voyeur nation? Changing definitions of voyeurism, 195-2004. Harv Rev Psychiatry. 2004;12:127–31.
3. Rye BJ, Meaney GJ. Voyeurism: it is good as long as we do not get caught. Int J Sex Health. 2007;19:47–56.

4. Downing L. Heteronormality and repronormality in sexological "perversion theory" and the DSM-5's "paraphilic disorder" diagnoses. Arch Sex Behav. 2015;44:1139–45.
5. Aggrawal A. References to the paraphilias and sexual crimes in the Bible. J Forensic Leg Med. 2009;16:109–14.
6. Smith RS. Voyeurism: a review of literature. Arch Sex Behav. 1976;5:585–608.
7. Lavin M. Voyeurism. Psychopathology and theory. In: Laws DR, O'Donohue WT, editors. Sexual deviance. Theory, assessment, and treatment. 2nd ed. New York: Guilford; 2008. p. 305–19.
8. Mann RE, Ainsworth F, Al-Attar Z, Davies M. Voyeurism. Assessment and treatment. In: Laws DR, O'Donohue WT, editors. Sexual deviance. Theory, assessment, and treatment. 2nd ed. New York: Guilford; 2008. p. 320–35.
9. Laws DR, O'Donohue WT, editors. Sexual deviance. Theory, assessment, and treatment. Second edition. New York: Guilford; 2008.
10. American Psychiatric Association. Diagnostic and statistical manual of mental disorders. 3rd ed. Washington, DC: American Psychiatric Association; 1980. p. 272–3.
11. American Psychiatric Association. Diagnostic and statistical manual of mental disorders. 5th ed. Arlington: American Psychiatric Association; 2013.
12. Jackson BT. A case of voyeurism treated by counterconditioning. Behav Res Ther. 1969;7:133–4.
13. Balon R. Controversies in the diagnosis and treatment of paraphilias. J Sex Marital Ther. 2013;39:7–20.
14. Emmanuel NP, Lydiard RB, Ballenger JC. Fluoxetine treatment of voyeurism. Am J Psychiatry. 1991;148:950.
15. Bianchi MD. Fluoxetine treatment of exhibitionism. Am J Psychiatry. 1990;147:1089–90.
16. Abouesh A, Clayton A. Compulsive voyeurism and exhibitionism: a clinical response to paroxetine. Arch Sex Behav. 1999;28:23–30.
17. Krueger RB, Kaplan MS. Depot-leuprolide acetate for treatment of paraphilias: a report of twelve cases. Arch Sex Behav. 2001;30:409–22.
18. Bradford JMW. The treatment of sexual deviation using a pharmacological approach. J Sex Res. 2000;37:248–57.
19. Bradford JMW. The neurobiology, neuropharmacology, and pharmacological treatment of the paraphilias and compulsive sexual behavior. Can J Psychiatry. 2001;46:26–34.

Chapter 6
Exhibitionistic Disorder

Richard Balon

As pointed out by Blair and Lanyon [1], there have been numerous attempts to define exhibitionism. At the time of their review [1], they noted that "All definitions involve the exposure to others of male genitalia, particularly the penis, at times and places that are considered interpersonally inappropriate. The element of sexual relevance and direct or indirect sexual gratification for the exhibitionist are usually, though not always, indicated or implied. Definitions differ on whether erection must be present" ([1], pp 439–440). Though exhibitionism/exhibitionistic disorder is, as most paraphilias/paraphilic disorders are, infrequent among females, the modern era diagnostic criteria are gender-neutral and use the general term of exposing one's genitalia to an unsuspecting subject. Thus psychiatry, sexuology, and sexual medicine conceptualize exhibitionism (and exhibitionistic disorder) in terms of what DSM-5 ([2], p 689) describes as "recurrent and

R. Balon, M.D. (✉)
Department of Psychiatry and Behavioral Neurosciences, Wayne State University, Tolan Park Building, 3rd Floor, 3901 Chrysler Service Dr., Detroit, MI 48201, USA

Department of Anesthesiology, Wayne State University, Tolan Park Building, 3rd Floor, 3901 Chrysler Service Dr., Detroit, MI 48201, USA
e-mail: rbalon@wayne.edu

R. Balon (ed.), *Practical Guide to Paraphilia and Paraphilic Disorders*, DOI 10.1007/978-3-319-42650-1_6

intense sexual fantasies from the exposure of one's genitals to an unsuspecting person, as manifested by fantasies, urges, or behaviors."

Similar to voyeurism/voyeuristic disorder (see Chap. 5), the concept of exhibitionism/exhibitionistic disorder in psychiatry and sexual medicine is more narrow than the general term of voyeurism, and carefully defined. Exhibitionism in terms of a disorder was described by French physician and psychiatrist Charles Lasegue in 1977 ([3], cited in [4]). However, cases of exposing one's genitalia or oneself naked have been described through the history, e.g., in the Bible [4], or in the case of Lady Godiva (which was not really a case of exhibitionism but rather a protest against taxation!). According to Langstrom [5], following voyeuristic behavior, exhibitionistic acts are among the most common of potentially law-breaking sexual behaviors, judging from clinical and general population samples. A number of descriptive studies of exhibitionism were done during the 1950s, 1960s, and 1970s [1]. Some of these studies used large samples of sexual offenders from courts, state hospitals, and forensic clinics. More recent research of exhibitionism/exhibitionistic disorder has been rather limited. Langstrom [5] hypothesizes that it is perhaps reflecting a long-standing perception that exhibitionistic behaviors are merely a nuisance compared to other sexual offenses. In addition, some exhibitionistic behaviors have become, if not acceptable, then at least more tolerated.

There are various types of exposure that maybe classified as exhibitionism, yet are not necessarily considered exhibitionism in the narrow psychiatry/sexual medicine terms. These include (a) anasyrma: the lifting of one's skirt when not wearing underwear; (b) candaulism: sexual practice or fantasy in which a man exposes his female partner, or images of her, to other people for their sexual pleasure; (c) flashing: the momentary display of bare breasts by a woman with an up-and-down lifting of the shirt and/or bra; or a brief exposure of female or male genitalia; (d) martymachlia—sexual attraction to having others watching the execution of a sexual act (at times, martymachlia is considered a paraphilia on its own);

(e) mooning: the display of bare buttocks by pulling down clothing—however, this is frequently done as an act of protest, mockery, or joke and not for sexual arousal purposes; (f) reflectoporn: the act of stripping and taking a picture of oneself using an object with a reflective surface as a mirror, then posting the image on the Internet in a public forum; and (g) streaking: the act of running naked through a public place—however, here again the intent is not usually sexual, but rather for shock value (retrieved mostly from Wikipedia on 2/29/2016). The newest type of exposure is called cyberflashing. It includes sending a picture of one's genitalia (mostly penis) to an unsuspecting person via AirDrop on one's smartphone (the sender is unknown to the person); or sending this picture to a still unsuspecting but known person (after a date or business meeting).

However, Blair and Lanyon [1] cautioned that the inappropriate interpersonal situations of genitalia exposure involve various exclusions, such as mutual sexual intimacy exposure (exposure may be limited by religious or cultural customs), medical examination exposure, or nudism or other forms of nonsexualized social nudity such as nude sunbathing or female partial nude sunbathing (topless). Last but not least, public urination should be also excluded [1].

The word exhibitionism has also been used in colloquial language for describing histrionics and showy or theatrical behavior. In addition to defining exhibitionism in terms of a tendency to expose one's genitalia, dictionaries such as Oxford's or Webster's define exhibitionism as a tendency to call attention to oneself or show off one's talent or skills; a behavior intended to attract attention to oneself.

Diagnostic Criteria

The core symptomatology of exhibitionism is the recurrent and intense arousal from the exposure of one's genitals to an unsuspecting person, manifested by fantasies, urges, and/or behaviors for a certain period of time, usually 6 months.

The DSM-5 [2] diagnosis of exhibitionistic disorder requires that the perpetrator has either acted on his/her urges with a nonconsenting person, or that these fantasies and urges caused him/her a clinically significant distress or impairment.

The criteria have developed and became more refined over time. The DSM-III [6] criteria for exhibitionism are fairly simple: "Repetitive acts of exposing the genitals to an unsuspecting stranger for the purpose of achieving sexual excitement, with no attempt at further sexual activity with the stranger." There was no defined period of time for the symptomatology to occur. The DSM-III-R [7] added the time period (6 months) for symptoms to occur and also added Criterion B, same for all paraphilias: "The person has acted on these urges, or is markedly distressed by them." Then DSM-IV [8] became more specific and closer to the recent criteria—Criterion A specified that "Over the period of at least 6 months, recurrent, intense sexually arousing fantasies, sexual urges, or behaviors involving the exposure of one's genitals to an unsuspecting stranger"; and Criterion B, "The fantasies, sexual urges, or behaviors cause clinically significant distress or impairment in social, occupational or other important areas of functioning." It is important to note that the DSM-IV removed from Criterion B the statement that the person "has acted on these urges." This change became confusing [5] and thus this statement was added back in subsequent editions of DSM [2, 9].

The DSM-5 Criteria of exhibitionistic disorder ([2], p 698) are as follows (Reprinted with permission from the Diagnostic and Statistical Manual of Mental Disorders, Fifth Edition, (Copyright 2013). American Psychiatric Association.):

Criterion A. Over a period of at least 6 months, recurrent and intense sexual arousal from the exposure of one's genitals to an unsuspecting person, as manifested by fantasies, urges, or behaviors.

Criterion B: The individual has acted on these sexual urges with a nonconsenting person, or the sexual urges or fantasies cause clinically significant distress or impairment in social, occupational, or other important areas of functioning.

Specify whether;
Sexually aroused by exposing genitals to prepubertal children

Sexually aroused by exposing genitals to physically mature individuals
Sexually aroused by exposing genitals to prepubertal children and to physically mature individuals

Specify:
In controlled environment: This specifier is primarily applicable to individuals living in institutional or other settings where opportunities to engage in voyeuristic behavior are restricted.

In full remission: The individual has not acted on the urges with a nonconsenting person, and there has been no distress or impairment in social, occupational or other areas of functioning, for at least 5 years while in an uncontrolled environment.

There are several caveats regarding the DSM-5 criteria. Understandably, the DSM-III [6] statement "with no attempt at further sexual activity with the stranger," was included to clarify that the act of exposing one's genitalia was the source final source of sexual excitement, as attempt at further sexual activity would mean rape. However, the DSM-III [6] language specifying that the purpose of exhibitionistic behavior was achieving sexual excitement disappeared. It is usually understood that the perpetrator of exhibitionistic behavior masturbates during or after the exposure or fantasizes about masturbating. The behavior is perpetrated with a non-consenting person, thus striptease is not exhibitionism. The DSM-5 ([2], pp 689–690) cautions that, "The diagnostic criteria for exhibitionistic disorder can apply both to individuals who more or less freely disclose this paraphilia and to those who categorically deny any sexual attraction to exposing their genitals to unsuspecting persons despite substantial objective evidence to the contrary. …Examples of nondisclosing individuals include those who have exposed themselves repeatedly to unsuspecting persons on separate occasions but who deny any urges or fantasies about such sexual behavior and who report that known episodes of exposure were all accidental and nonsexual." The DSM-5 also defines recurrent genital exposures as three or more victims on separate occasions, and that recurrent could also mean fewer victims of exposure if there were multiple exposures to the same victim.

Murphy and Page [10] pointed out that exhibitionists frequently engage in a variety of other paraphilic behaviors, such as voyeurism, frottage, and even rape. Thus, there could be a significant overlap among exhibitionism/exhibitionistic disorder and other paraphilias. Others [11] reported that a significant portion of exhibitionists also molested children. Many exhibitionists have been also arrested for nonsexual offenses [1].

Summary of Evidence

As with other paraphilias, the true incidence and prevalence of exhibitionism are unknown [10] (I am discussing prevalence/incidence of exhibitionism, not of exhibitionistic disorder, as the diagnosis of exhibitionistic disorder is new and has not been used in any studies estimating the prevalence and/or incidence). Nevertheless, the DSM-5 [2] cites the highest possible prevalence for exhibitionistic disorder (sic!) in males to be 2–4 %, based on exhibitionistic acts in nonclinical or general populations. Langstrom and Seto [12] in a Swedish National Population Survey found the lifetime prevalence of any episode of exhibitionistic disorder to be 4.1 % for men and 2.1 % for women (3.1 % of responders in that survey admitted to exhibitionistic acts for sexual pleasure). Murphy and Page [10] noted that criminal justice data, victim surveys, and limited community surveys suggest that exhibitionism occurs frequently (whatever frequently means here). In their analysis, one-third to one-half of all sexual crimes reported to police in some countries were acts of exhibitionism. They added that reports to police clearly underestimate the prevalence and incidence. Murphy and Page [10] also cite estimates from some community samples in the UK, but these samples were too small for any meaningful conclusion. The prevalence of exhibitionism in females is believed to be much lower, but is truly unknown (especially considering the various degrees of exposing oneself mentioned earlier). In summary, the prevalence of exhibitionism seems to be relatively high, especially when compared to other paraphilias.

The age of onset of exhibitionistic behavior is usually in the early to mid-20s, tough possibly also in adolescence [1]. According to the DSM-5 [2], males with exhibitionistic behavior usually become aware of their interest in exposing their genitals to unsuspecting persons during their adolescence. The DSM-5 [2] also notes that it may be difficult to differentiate between age-appropriate sexual curiosity in adolescents and true exhibitionistic behaviors. The course of exhibitionism/exhibitionistic disorder is unknown, i.e., probably varies with age [2] and may decrease with advanced age [2].

Langstrom and Seto [12] found that those reporting exhibitionistic, but not voyeuristic, behavior were significantly younger, were more often separated from their parents, and were living in major urban areas. Most exhibitionists in various studies [1] were married, many of them happily. It seems that exhibitionists may be generally hypersexual [12, 13]. Antisocial personality disorder, alcohol use disorder, and pedophilic interest could be risk factors for exhibitionistic disorder/behavior in males with exhibitionistic interests [2]. Interestingly, in one recent study [14] approximately half of exhibitionistic incidents reported by victims of exhibitionism occurred on a subway train or platform and in a crowded place, contrary to the popular belief that these acts occur in parks, wooded areas, streets, or parking lots, not in crowded places. As the authors of this study (conducted in New York City) noted, previous studies on the locations of exhibitionistic acts were done in cities without a subway system. Exhibitionism together with voyeurism is the most common law-breaking sexual behaviors [5, 12].

Similar to other paraphilias/paraphilic disorders, the etiology of exhibitionism/exhibitionistic disorder is unknown. Psychodynamic theories were the first coherent attempts to explain exhibitionism. Castration anxiety has been frequently used as an explanatory framework—"The individual is said to exhibit to receive verification that his penis really does exist" ([1], p 448). The individual is thought to exhibit to young girls as he is afraid of castration by older, more mature women who may or may not resemble his mother [1].

It is important to note that there are no data to explain this theory [1]. Another prominent theory attempting to explain exhibitionism is the courtship theory postulated by Freund (e.g., [15, 16]). Exhibitionism could be viewed as a distortion or extreme intensification of the second, affiliative, phase of courtship which is normally characterized by nonverbal and verbal overtures such as looking at, smiling, and talking to a potential partner. Other attempts to explain exhibitionism include learning, behavioral, and biological theories. None of the theories has satisfactorily explained exhibitionism. The courtship theory seems the most plausible one, yet still just a theory.

The assessment of a person being evaluated for exhibitionism/exhibitionistic disorder starts with a clinical interview which is the cornerstone of the evaluation. The interview should be conducted in comfortable and trusting manner (depending on the environment/situation—clinical vs. forensic evaluation, private office vs. prison). If the patient acknowledges his/her exhibitionistic behavior, he/she should be asked how long and how often he/she has been engaged in this behavior, how he/she feels while and after exposing, and how he/she feels about the possibility of changing and regaining his/her life [17]. If possible, the initial evaluation should include corroborative information, preferably obtained in corroborative interviews (partner, family), and information from reviewing records (especially in criminal cases). Careful attention should be paid to comorbid paraphilias/paraphilic disorders and other psychiatric comorbidity.

There are no specific tests for exhibitionism/exhibitionistic disorder. Penile plethysmography has not yielded satisfactory results and is potentially more useful in assessing additional paraphilias other than exhibitionism itself [17]. In addition, as pointed out by Blair and Lanyon ([1], p 459), penile erections may not always be a viable measure in exhibitionism, since erection is not required for exhibitionism and can be also voluntarily suppressed even in the presence of sexual stimuli. Neuropsychological testing could be useful only in assessing cases of exhibitionism/exhibitionistic disorder with suspected organic etiology.

Treatment of exhibitionism/exhibitionistic disorder is a relatively uncharted area. Most of the recommendations regarding therapy are exhibitionism nonspecific, and discuss an all encompassing group of sex offenders. The earlier literature [1] was skeptical about the success of "verbal" therapies. Nevertheless, the newer literature recommends various therapies (again, if tested, then mostly for sex offenders in general). Group therapy has been used in institutionalized sex offenders and has been touted as cost effective and providing an opportunity to discuss the exhibitionistic activities in an atmosphere of accountability [17]. Cognitive-behavioral approaches focuses mostly on relapse prevention, and on working with intimacy deficit and boundaries. Relapse prevention is a very important and at times effective intervention. Morin and Levenson ([17], p 93) provide an excellent example of concrete relapse prevention strategy, which includes avoiding high-risk situations and introducing obstacles to the chain of events: "many exhibitionists expose themselves from their cars while driving. Such an offender may engage in grooming behaviors such as calling an unsuspecting victim over to the window to ask for directions, at which point the victim witnesses the offender exposing himself and masturbating. Such an offender can interfere with this pattern by removing the fuses for the powered windows in his car. Avoiding any unnecessary driving, and avoiding routes that present opportunities for offending may also be helpful." Behavioral approaches, such as covert sensitization and aversive techniques have also been suggested. Marshall [18] reported a case of a male exhibitionist who was given a small bottle of ammonia salts to smell whenever he had an urge to expose himself. It helped to decrease the urges. The urges finally stopped and in addition patient mood got better, more self-confident, and socially active.

Biological treatment modalities used in exhibitionism/exhibitionistic disorder include serotonergic antidepressants and hormones. They should be combined with cognitive-behavioral therapies and other therapies and should probably follow the algorithm outlined by Bradford [19] for treatment of paraphilias in general. There are a couple of reports of successful treatment of exhibitionism with SSRIs. Bianchi [20] administered fluoxetine up to 40 mg/day to a man diagnosed earlier with schizophrenia who complained of fantasies involving genital exposure. The fantasies were relieved by fluoxetine for the first time since early childhood. One of the three cases described by Perilstein, Lipper, and Friedman [21] was a 30-year-old man with a 7-year history of regular exhibitionism. Psychotherapy with psychodynamic and behavioral approaches was not consistently helpful and covert sensitization helped only temporarily. Thus, he was treated with fluoxetine 80 mg a day and his urges decreased. His sexual desire was decreased and ejaculation retarded, yet this did not interfere with his pleasurable sexual experience. His improvement was sustained on fluoxetine in 6-month follow-up. Abouesh and Clayton [22] described a case of a 29-year-old male who exposed himself to a woman at his home and reported recurring compulsive thoughts of exposing himself to women. He actually described being sexually aroused by a pretty woman, and then planning to lure her to a safe place and then expose himself to her. He was started on a low dose of paroxetine, which was gradually increased to 30 mg a day. He was able to resist his impulses and continued to do well for 2½ months till being lost to follow-up. A series of 12 paraphilia cases treated with leuprolide acetate by Kruger and Kaplan [23] included five patients with exhibitionism as at least one of their diagnoses (there was a significant degree of comorbidity with other paraphilias such as voyeurism, frotteurism, and other mental disorders). All of them responded to leuprolide acetate 7.5 mg or 3.75 mg intramuscularly at monthly intervals, were reporting markedly reduced sexual arousal and cessation of exhibitionistic behavior.

Clinical Example (Fictitious Case Made Up/Anonymized from Several Cases)

A 22-year-old male college student was referred for treatment after being arrested by police for his "deviant sexual offense exposing himself to a woman." He actually drove to a fast food restaurant drive-in line and ordered food. While picking up his food he exposed himself to a female cashier window worker and after she yelled at him he started to masturbate and drove away. The victim quickly noted his license plate in the window mirror and called the police. He was caught while still driving and arrested.

During the initial evaluation he admitted that this was not the first time he exposed himself. He has fantasized about exposing himself to women since his early adolescence. He actually exposed himself for the first time at the age of 17 at one of the city parks, when it was already dark. He was waiting close to one of the public lights and when he saw a female approaching, he dropped his pants a bit, exposed his penis to her and ran away. He masturbated later while fantasizing about this encounter. He said he has exposed himself to women "numerous times" at different parks around the metropolitan area. Lately, he started to prefer to expose himself while in the car. However, his exhibitionistic behavior at the drive through window was only his second one. He enjoyed the thrill of exposing himself very much and frequently masturbated at home while fantasizing about having sex with his victims.

He also revealed that as a young boy he loved to watch women undressing through the windows of apartments in a complex where his family lived. "That stopped to be interesting once I started to expose myself, exposing has been much more thrilling and arousing."

He attended college where he studied business and Spanish, planning to get an MBA and work "somewhere in Latin America, life is easier there, women are friendlier and more accessible." He has dated several female students on the campus, usually for a brief period of time. He has been sexually active with his girlfriends, but "exposing has been more exciting."

He denied any other problem except for binge drinking. He denied being intoxicated when exposing himself.

He was very worried that the university would find out about his sexual offense and that he would be expelled. His parents were very supportive and helped him find a psychiatrist. He was awaiting trial for his sexual offense and was keen to start treatment as soon as possible. As he has already been in therapy with a cognitive-behavioral therapist, he wanted to add medication "to help me to get rid of my urges completely." After the discussion of medication options—SSRIs vs. hormonal therapy, it was decided to start him on paroxetine. The dose was gradually titrated up to 80 mg a day, in addition to CBT. His urges ceased and he has not been exposing himself. He has been in treatment for 4 years and continues to do well, with no episodes of exhibitionistic behavior or urges to expose himself. He has been in a stable relationship.

Recommendations

Patients with suspected or confirmed exhibitionism/exhibitionistic disorder should be carefully evaluated to determine the presence of exhibitionistic behavior, its frequency and presence of distress or impairment in various areas of functioning. A detailed clinical interview should be the cornerstone of the initial evaluation. The approach to the patient should be nonjudgmental, empathic. The evaluation should focus on urges, fantasies, behaviors, and also on overlap with other paraphilias/paraphilic disorders (e.g., pedophilic disorder) and other mental disorders (e.g., personality disorders and substance use disorders). Thus, the evaluating clinician should appreciate whether the patient prefers exposing genitals to prepubertal children, physically mature adults, or both. The clinical interview should also focus on issues such as hypersexuality and compulsivity of the exhibitionistic behavior, sexual fantasy content, beliefs about deviance/harm to others, self-esteem, impact on relationships and social functioning, anxiety, depression, and substance abuse.

Similar to the treatment of other paraphilias/paraphilic disorders, the treatment of exhibitionism/exhibitionistic disorder should start with developing a therapeutic relationship and an atmosphere of trust. Clinicians may follow the algorithm proposed by Bradford [19]. Therapy, namely CBT, relapse-prevention, covert sensitization, and even aversion approaches should be the first step in the management of this disorder. As Morin and Levenson [17] emphasized, many sex offenders, including exhibitionists, display intimacy deficits and dysfunctional styles of attachment, and have also experienced a number of boundary violations during their development that distorted the acquisition of healthy boundaries. Thus, therapy should also address these issues, in addition to identifying the emotional needs of exhibitionists and carefully address them. The use of other therapy modalities, e.g., group therapy, social skills training, or even 12-step programs for persons with sexual addiction, should be explored. Patients may also be referred local chapters of programs such as Sexaholics Anonymous, and recommended to read some self-help books.

SSRIs such as fluoxetine and paroxetine should be added if there is no improvement. The doses used may be relatively high in an effort to suppress the sexual urges. Hormonal therapy (medroxyprogesterone acetate, cyproterone acetate, flutamide, triptorelin, leuprolide acetate, goserelin acetate) should be reserved for cases resistant to SSRIs and psychotherapy, for cases of recidivism and for cases encompassing several paraphilias/paraphilic disorders, especially those causing more harm to others, e.g., sadistic disorder or pedophilic disorder. Combining various treatments seems prudent, though there is no evidence addressing treatment combinations. Treatment risks and side effects should always be discussed with the patient, even in cases of court-mandated treatment.

References

1. Blair DC, Lanyon RI. Exhibitionism: etiology and treatment. Psychol Bull. 1981;89:439–63.
2. American Psychiatric Association. Diagnostic and statistical manual of mental disorders. 5th ed. Arlington: American Psychiatric Association; 2013.
3. Lasegue C. Les exhibitionistes. L'Union Medicale (Paris). 1877;series 3; 23:709–14.
4. Aggrawal A. References to the paraphilias and sexual crimes in the Bible. J Forensic Leg Med. 2009;16:109–14.
5. Langstrom N. The DSM diagnostic criteria for exhibitionism, voyeurism, and frotteurism. Arch Sex Behav. 2010;39:317–24.
6. American Psychiatric Association. Diagnostic and statistical manual of mental disorders. 3rd ed. Washington, DC: American Psychiatric Association; 1980. p. 272.
7. American Psychiatric Association. Diagnostic and statistical manual of mental disorders. 3rd ed., rev. Washington, DC: American Psychiatric Association; 1987. p. 282.
8. American Psychiatric Association. Diagnostic and statistical manual of mental disorders. 4th ed. Washington, DC: American Psychiatric Association; 1994. p. 526.
9. American Psychiatric Association. Diagnostic and statistical manual of mental disorders. 4th ed., text rev. Washington, DC: American Psychiatric Association; 2000.
10. Murphy WD, Page IJ. Exhibitionism. Psychopathology and theory. In: Laws DR, O'Donohue WT, editors. Sexual deviance. Theory, assessment, and treatment. 2nd ed. New York: Guilford; 2008. p. 61–75.
11. Abel G, Osborn C. Stopping sexual violence. Psychiatric Ann. 1992;22:301–6.
12. Langstrom N, Seto MC. Exhibitionistic and voyeuristic behavior in a Swedish National Population Survey. Arch Sex Behav. 2006;35:427–35.
13. Kafka MP, Hennen J. Hypersexual desire in males: are males with paraphilias different from males with paraphilia-related disorders? Sex Abuse. 2003;15:307–21.
14. Clark SK, Jeglic EL, Calkins C, Tatar JR. More than a nuisance: the prevalence and consequences of frotteurism and exhibitionism. Sex Abuse. 2016;28:3–19.

15. Freund K, Watson R. Mapping the boundaries of courtship disorder. J Sex Res. 1990;27:589–606.
16. Freund K, Seto MC. Preferential rape in the theory of courtship disorder. Arch Sex Behav. 1998;27:433–43.
17. Morin JW, Levenson JS. Exhibitionism. Assessment and treatment. In: Laws DR, O'Donohue WT, editors. Sexual deviance. Theory, assessment, and treatment. 2nd ed. New York: Guilford; 2008. p. 76–107.
18. Marshall WL. Ammonia aversion with an exhibitionist: a case study. Clin Case Stud. 2005;5:15–24.
19. Bradford JMW. The neurobiology, neuropharmacology, and pharmacological treatment of the paraphilias and compulsive sexual behavior. Can J Psychiatry. 2001;46:26–34.
20. Bianchi MD. Fluoxetine reatment of exhibitionism. Am J Psychiatry. 1990;147:1089–90.
21. Perilstein RD, Lipper S, Friendman LJ. Three cases if paraphilias responsive to fluoxetine treatment. J Clin Psychiatry. 1991;52:169–70.
22. Abouesh A, Clayton A. Compulsive voyeurism and exhibitionism: a clinical response to paroxetine. Arch Sex Behav. 1999;28:23–30.
23. Kruger RB, Kaplan MS. Depot-leuprolide acetate for treatment of paraphilias: a report of twelve cases. Arch Sex Behav. 2001;30:409–22.

Chapter 7
Frotteuristic Disorder

Richard Balon

Frotteurism/frotteuristic disorder seems to be a fairly rare paraphilia/paraphilic disorder, as attested not only by its relatively low prevalence (though estimates vary, see below in the Summary of evidence section), but mainly by the lack of data about it in the literature. Interestingly, the DSM-III [1] did not include frotteurism among its 8 paraphilias listed with diagnostic criteria. Frotteurism first appeared in the DSM-III-R [2], basically replacing zoophilia in the list of paraphilias with DSM diagnostic criteria. Frotteuristic disorder is included in DSM-5 [3].

The use and meaning of the word frotteurism in sexual terms originated with a French psychiatrist Valentin Magnan in 1890 ([4], cited in [5]). He described men committing an act of what he called frottage—rubbing an exposed penis against the buttocks of unsuspecting women. The word frottage comes from the French "frotter," which means to rub or to put pres-

R. Balon, M.D. (✉)
Department of Psychiatry and Behavioral Neurosciences, Wayne State University, Tolan Park Building, 3rd Floor, 3901 Chrysler Service Dr., Detroit, MI 48201, USA

Department of Anesthesiology, Wayne State University, Tolan Park Building, 3rd Floor, 3901 Chrysler Service Dr., Detroit, MI 48201, USA
e-mail: rbalon@wayne.edu

R. Balon (ed.), *Practical Guide to Paraphilia and Paraphilic Disorders*, DOI 10.1007/978-3-319-42650-1_7

sure on someone, and has no sexual connotation [5]. Frotteur means the "one who rubs." The word was incorporated into sexuology terminology and popularized by Richard von Kraft-Ebbing in his seminal book [6]. A frotteuristic act in contemporary thinking means deriving intense sexual arousal from touching or rubbing, usually one's genitals (penis) or pelvic area against a non-consenting person. The diagnostic criteria (see below) are fairly nonspecific about what touching and rubbing exactly means. Over the years, there has been some disagreement about whether frotteurism has to really include rubbing genitals against an unsuspecting person [5]. Some have argued that frotteurism does not need to include the perpetrator's genitals and that the act of frotteurism should also include sexual urges to touch and acts of touching. Thus the recent view includes both rubbing and touching as part of a frotteuristic act. Others also argued that toucherism—sexual arousal derived from touching, grabbing, or rubbing one's hand against an unsuspecting person's areas such as crotch and breasts—should be included. The DSM-III-R [2] specifies that its category of frotteurism includes both frotteurism and toucherism. A bit vague DSM-5 terminology basically implies the same.

As noted by Clark and colleagues [7], frotteurism/frotteuristic disorder is one of the least understood types of paraphilias/paraphilic disorders listed in our classifications. This is partially due to the fact that a lot of what is known about this disorder has been extracted from studies focused on other paraphilias, namely exhibitionism [7]. The act of frotteurism happens in crowded places, subway trains and platforms [7], busy sidewalks [2], escalators, elevators, shopping places, and theatres. The perpetrator thus has an opportunity to disappear in the crowd and escape arrest. The act of frotteurism frequently is not reported by the victims. Some reasons for underreporting frotteurism may be the fact that the victims may not be fully aware of the act in a crowded place, or do not recognize the act or the perpetrator (the encounter may not be face-to-face and may be without verbal exchange). The perpetrator may also claim that what happened was an accidental encounter due to the crowded place. In addition, frotteurism has been frequently considered a nuisance crime

[7, 8] by the legal system and thus not investigated and prosecuted as frequently as some other paraphilias/paraphilic disorders. Of note: Clark and colleagues [7] correctly argue that frotteurism should not be considered just a nuisance crime, as a number of the victims in their study reported negative consequences of victimization such as feelings of violation and changes of behavior.

Popular media have reported that frotteurism is "widespread" in some countries, e.g., India and Japan. Reportedly, in Japan there are some trains and buses with women-only spaces to decrease the opportunity for men to perpetrate the act of frotteurism. There is a special Japanese term—chikan—for public molestation, or for the person who commits such an act, e.g., groping on crowded trains. The act of frotteurism is said to be more tolerated in Japan. However, scientific literature in English is lacking (and there is only one article in Japanese on this topic I am aware of—[9]).

As noted, the literature on frotteurism is scarce. Similar to other paraphilias/paraphilic disorders, a lot of guidance on managing frotteurism/frotteuristic disorder is based on scarce evidence and assumptions.

Diagnostic Criteria

The core element of touching or rubbing against a nonconsenting person has been part of the DSM classification in some variations since the time of its appearance in DSM-III-R [2]. The DSM-III-R did not include "behaviors" in Criterion A. On the other hand, DSM-III-R [2] was specific about what is sexually exciting. It stated (p 284) that "It is the touching, not the coercive nature of the act that is sexually exciting."

The DSM-5 criteria of frotteuristic disorder ([3], pp 691–692) are as follows (Reprinted with permission from the Diagnostic and Statistical Manual of Mental Disorders, Fifth Edition, (Copyright 2013). American Psychiatric Association) are as follows:

> *Criterion A. Over the period of at least 6 months, recurrent and intense sexual arousal from touching or rubbing against a nonconsenting person, as manifested by fantasies, urges or behaviors.*

Criterion B. The individual has acted on these sexual urges with a nonconsenting person, or the sexual urges or fantasies cause clinically significant distress or impairment in social, occupational, or other important areas of functioning.

Specify:
In controlled environment: This specifier is primarily applicable to individuals living in institutional or other settings where opportunities to engage in voyeuristic behavior are restricted.

In full remission: The individual has not acted on the urges with a nonconsenting person, and there has been no distress or impairment in social, occupational or other areas of functioning, for at least 5 years while in an uncontrolled environment.

The DSM-5 specifies that the diagnostic criteria of frotteuristic disorder can be applied both to individuals who fairly freely disclose their frotteuristic behavior, and to those who firmly deny any sexual attraction derived from frotteuristic acts regardless of objective experience to the contrary.

Lussier and Piche [5] pointed out some weaknesses of the diagnostic criteria of frotteurism/frotteuristic disorder, including a possible overlap with other paraphilia/paraphilic disorders. One such weakness is the lack of specifications about the victim—they asked ([5], p 133), "…if the rubbing or touching involves prepubescent boys or girls, should it be conceived as indicative of frotteurism, pedophilia or both?" Similarly, the description of the behavior is not totally clear, thus they ([5], p 133) ask again "…if the behavior involves exposure of the genitals, should it be conceived as indicative of frotteurism, exhibitionism, or even fetishism?" The last important point that Lussier and Piche ([5], p 133) made is about the context of frotteuristic act. It is important to remember that "sexual excitement from fondling ant touching one's sexual partner is part of normal sexual activity" and thus "it must be kept in mind that a central aspect of making frotteurism a paraphilia is the *context* in which the behavior occurs" (i.e., in contrast to some other paraphilias/paraphilic behavior, it is not the act itself that is deviant, but the fact that it involves a nonconsenting person).

An interesting point about frotteurism was raised by Horley [10]. He suggested that the diagnostic criteria of this paraphilia are imprecise. He suggested that frotteurism may be viewed as an ineffectual sexual assault and "frotteurs" as less aggressive or timid rapists (i.e., they may commit more serious assault in different circumstances, such as if the victim would be very submissive). This, according to Horley [10] would eliminate the need for a separate diagnostic category of frotteurism/frotteuristic disorder. However, as Langstrom argued, we lack data to either support or reject this suggestion [11].

The diagnostic category of frotteurism/frotteuristic disorder clearly desires more research and data to clarify whether this entity should be separated from other paraphilias/paraphilic disorders and continued as a separate disorder. If frotteurism/ frotteuristic disorder is continued to be conceptualized as a separate diagnostic entity, further clarification and more specific criteria are needed, including some specifications about the victims (age?).

Summary of Evidence

The estimates of prevalence of frotteurism/frotteuristic disorder prevalence vary widely. DSM-5 suggests that frotteuristic acts (touching or rubbing) may occur in up to 30 % of adult males in the general population. Johnson and colleagues [12] in their systematic review of prevalence of this paraphilia/ paraphilic disorder found four studies in which the prevalence of frotteurism in men varied from 7 to 9.1, 9.7, and 35 %. They felt that these studies were of limited methodological quality and that the estimates varied for reasons such as not excluding childhood behavior in the study with the highest estimate, to inconsistent method of asking questions about the act, its frequency, etc. Clark and colleagues [7] wrote that reliable estimates of prevalence are difficult to obtain. According to them, official reports are likely to underestimate the frequency of frotteurism, as the acts are infrequently brought to the attention of authorities, and the perpetrators themselves tend to under-report their behavior especially in the criminal system setting. The estimates may also differ in different population samples. For instance, Abel and colleagues [13] in their study of 561 non-incarcerated sex offenders found the prevalence of frotteuristic behavior to be 25 %. On the other hand, Becker and colleagues [14] in their study of a group of sex offenders residing in a facility for civilly committed sex offenders found that 5 % of the offenders had a diagnosis of frotteurism. Clark and colleagues [7] suggested that given the fairly high number of victims per perpetrator (e.g., [13]), high rate of median paraphilic acts (29.5, cited in [15]) and the low incidence of reporting, a more accurate way of assessing the frequency of occurrence may be using victim self-report. The results of their study indicated a fairly high rate of victimization among female college students—approximately 24 % of women in their sample (and 8 % of men) reported having been a victim of frotteuristic behavior at least once in their lifetime (comparable numbers for exhibitionism were 40 % of women and 12 % men). The mentioned media reports from countries such as Japan and India also suggest that a frotteuristic act may be a crime of opportunity. Obviously, the exact prevalence of frotteurism/frotteuristic disorder in the general population is unknown and quite difficult to estimate. However, the rate of victims of frotteurism may be fairly high, especially in some populations and places, such as riders of public transportation. Thus, it is impossible to determine the overall prevalence of frotteurism/frotteuristic disorder in the general population.

The data regarding the age of onset of frotteurism/frotteuristic disorder are unclear. According to the DSM-5 ([3], p 693), males with frotteuristic disorder often report that they first became aware of their sexual interest in touching unsuspecting persons during late adolescence or emerging adulthood. However, children may also touch or rub against an unwilling person in the absence of frotteurism. The DSM-5 also notes that frotteuristic disorder may be difficult to differentiate from conduct-disordered behavior without sexual motivation in younger individuals. Some studies reported the age of onset being fairly early (10-12 years [16]), while Abel and Osborne [15] cite the age of onset to be 20.7 years or 29.5 years, depending on the source. Lussier and Piche [5] speculated that on average frotteurism tends to start in early adulthood, i.e., at a relatively later stage of the development of sexual deviance over time.

Not much is known about the characteristics of persons with frotteurism/frotteuristic disorder, and the course of this paraphilic disorder. The estimates of the frequency of frotteuristic acts vary widely and the persistence of this behavior over time is not clear [3]. Persons suffering from frotteurism/froteturistic disorder are frequently involved in antisocial activities. The course is likely to vary with time, and similar to some other paraphilis/paraphilic disorders, the sexual preferences and behaviors may decline with older age [3].

Like in the case of other paraphilias/paraphilic disorders, the etiology of frotteurism/froteturistic disorder is unknown. Several theoretical models of etiology of frotteurism have been proposed. One of them is the courtship disorders theory [17, 18] with its description of behavioral interactions leading to sexual intercourse (finding, affiliative, tactile, and copulatory phases). Frotteurism/frotteuristic behavior is a distortion of the tactile phase, in which physical contact is made. Lussier and Piche [5] also mention other theories, such as the social incompetence hypothesis (the elements would probably include shyness, inhibition, uncertainty about virility in the presence of women) and the sex drive hypothesis (the inability to control sex drive). Lussier and Piche ([5], p 141) found no supporting evidence for the latter theory. Lussier and Piche ([5], p 141)) also raised an interesting point that the fact that a substantial proportion of young adults self-report unwanted sexual touching and rubbing suggests that severe psychological impairment is not necessary for this behavior to occur. That again, like in many paraphilias, blurs the distinction between what is "normal" (whatever it means in this discussion) and what is pathological, and suggests a continuum or spectrum of this behavior. It is important to note that frotteuristic acts can also occur in individuals with intellectual disabilities, in some neurodevelopmental disorders (e.g., autism spectrum disorders), in cases of other brain/organic disorders, e.g., Parkinson's disease, and medications being used to treat these diseases. Cannas and colleagues [19] described a case of a 51-year-old male with Parkinson's disease who after years of treatment with a dopaminergic medication pergolide developed frotteurism and delusional jealousy. Both the frotteuristic behavior and jealousy ceased after pergolide was decreased and quetiapine added. These cases should be evaluated very carefully to make a distinction between true frotteurism/frotteuristic disorder and symptoms that are part of an uncontrolled behavior within the frame of these disorders. The differential diagnosis considerations should also include substance use disorders, and conduct and antisocial personality disorders.

The main elements of the assessment of an individual with suspected or confirmed frotteurism/frotteuristic behavior are a comprehensive clinical interview, collateral information (from victims, authorities such as police or other legal authorities, and family) and complementary documentation (from authorities, previous evaluations, and other health care professionals). The evaluation should be conducted, as much as possible, in an atmosphere of trust (depending on the environment/situation—clinical vs. forensic evaluation, private office vs. prison). There are no specific tests for diagnosing frotteurism/frotteuristic disorder. Various scales and tests such as the Minnesota Multiple Personality Inventory can be used, but only for the assessment of comorbid psychopathology and not for the assessment of frotteurism. Penile phaloplethysmography is not useful for evaluation of frotteurism/frotteuristic disorder.

The literature on treatment of this disorder is really scarce. As Johnson and colleagues [12] pointed out, there are no studies on the treatment of frotteurism. Kuruvilla and Joseph [20] described a case of a 50-year-old man who complained of seminal emissions when he came into contact with any part of the body of another man—whenever he rubbed against another man, he indulged in pleasurable homosexual fantasies culminating in ejaculation. His treatment started with systematic desensitization that decreased anxiety, but not his frotteuristic behavior. In the next stage of treatment, aversive therapy for frotteuristic behavior was introduced. Interestingly, low voltage but painful electrical shock was used, however it is not clear whether it was not just part of the imagery. This case raises ethical questions as it also included cessation of homosexual fantasies following the aversion therapy.

One of the three cases of paraphilias responding to fluoxetine in a report by Perilstein, Lipper, and Friedman [21] was a man suffering from voyuerism and frotteurism. He responded well to 20 mg of fluoxetine a day and continued doing well in a 3-month follow-up. Patra and colleagues [22] reported a case of hypersexual frotteuristic behavior in an individual who was also diagnosed with comorbid depression. He responded well to sertraline 100 mg/day and clonazepam 0.25 mg at bedtime, along with supportive therapy. The behavior (and depression) gradually ceased over the period of 4–6 weeks and he did well in 6-months follow-up. However, the individual in this case was a 12-year-old boy and thus it is difficult to ascertain whether this was really a case of frotteurism within the framework of our diagnostic system (though the DSM system does not specify an age of onset for frotteurism/frotteuristic disorder). Kalra [23] presented a case of a 25-year-old man who indulged in genital rubbing against women on trains (he would switch trains if no suitable victim found on a train). Interestingly, on a few occasions he also went with 9–10 men to indulge in group genital rubbing against women in the crowd (they even had a local term for this activity, "tekaa bharna"). As the patient was totally preoccupied with this behavior and became distressed, he also became depressed. He sought professional help. He was started on fluoxetine 20 mg/day and the dose was gradually increased to 60 mg/day. His depression ceased and his sexual urges had reduced. He reported almost 80 % reduction in his genital rubbing over a period of 8 months. He was able to postpone acting out on his sexual urges. Finally, one of the 12 subjects in a report by Krueger and Kaplan [24] had a history of exhibitionism, frotteurism, voyeurism, public masturbation, psychotic disorder not otherwise specified, and multiple rapes of women. He was incarcerated and committed to a state mental health facility.

He reported continual preoccupation and sexual fantasy of raping and exposing himself to women. He did not respond to fluoxetine up to 80 mg/day. He was started on leuprolide acetate 7.5 mg intramuscularly at monthly intervals for 12 months. He reported a loss of all sexual functioning and his deviant fantasies and arousal. Leuprolide acetate was discontinued due to adverse effects such as unilateral gynecomastia and complete loss of sexual functioning. This was clearly a complicated case due to several coexisting disorders and thus the effect of leuprolide acetate on just frotteurism is difficult to assess.

Various therapeutic approaches have been touted [5] with cognitive-behavioral therapy being the most prominent. However, case reports or studies specific to frotteurism are missing in the literature.

Clinical Example (Fictitious Case with Material Used from Other Cases)

A 40-year-old male mechanic seeks help after one of his coworkers noted that he was rubbing his genitals against an unsuspecting woman's buttocks on a crowded bus. The coworker pressed the patient "to do something about it" as this was a second time he noticed while they were commuting to work on the same bus line. The coworker told him that if this is a recurrent issue then rather than being ultimately caught by police he should look for professional help. During the initial evaluation the patient revealed that he had been rubbing his genitals against women "with big buttocks" for a number of years. "I have been lucky that they usually do not notice, maybe they don't feel it that well, or maybe they enjoy it." He said that he had occasionally ejaculated during rubbing when his sexual tension was "high" or when "we were stuck in traffic for a long time." He admits that he occasionally tried to brush his hand against the breasts of women with "huge breasts." "But I stopped doing it as I almost got caught a couple of times. I had to run away fast."

The personal history revealed a shy, single man living alone. After graduation from high school he started to work as a mechanic and has been with the same company for all his adult life. He was fraternizing with colleagues at work, but did not have other friends. He dated "a few girls, I had sex with them, it was OK, but I like those women with huge buttocks and big breasts. I liked to press against my girls from the back before having sex." He was not exactly sure when he started to rub against unsuspecting women's bodies. "It started when I was much younger, maybe just out of high school." He admits that he would "get a drink or two before getting on the bus, there is a pub outside of our shop. Drinks help me to get into it, I am not anxious at all about it after a drink or two. Without them, I get a bit tense, nervous, but I still enjoy it." He has never talked about his frotteuristic acts with anybody. He was relieved that his colleague has not talked to anybody else, as "the guys in the shop would really make fun of me."

He refused to be on medication, "I read about medications on the Internet, they kill your pleasure, I don't want it." He started to see a therapist and CBT was initiated. He reported "being better, I am staying away from it." However, he stopped participating in CBT after 2 months and was lost to follow-up.

Recommendations

Patients with suspected or confirmed frotteurism/frotteuristic disorder should be carefully evaluated to determine the presence of frotteuristic behavior, its frequency and the presence of distress or impairment in various areas of functioning. A detailed clinical interview should be the cornerstone of the initial evaluation. The approach to the patient should be nonjudgmental, empathic. The evaluation should focus on urges, fantasies, behaviors, and also on overlap with other paraphilias/paraphilic disorders (e.g., voyeuristic and exhibitionistic disorders), other mental disorders (e.g., personality disorders and substance use disorders), and even physical/neurological disorders and their treatment (e.g., Parkinsonism, dopaminergic medications).

As with other paraphilias/paraphilic disorders the treatment of frotteurism/frotteuristic disorder should start with developing a therapeutic relationship and an atmosphere of trust. Supportive and/or cognitive behavioral therapy should probably be the first line of treatment. The patients may be given self-help texts (Sexaholics Anonymous White Book). They may be referred to programs such as Sexaholics Anonymous, Sex and Love Addicts Anonymous, or Sex Addicts Anonymous (local chapters may be found online). They should be recommended to try several different meetings in different locations if possible, to find one that fits them most [5]. They should be advised that there is no frotteurism specific program available, so that they would not be discouraged during the first few visits.

Medication should be tried if there is no improvement, or right away in combination with therapy in more severe cases. Serotonergic antidepressants (SSRIs and clomipramine) should be tried first among medications, though there is no clear guidance as to what to do in cases of frotteurism/frotteuristic disorder. One may try to use the algorithm proposed by Bradford [25] as a guidance though it has not been reported to be tested in this indication.

Hormonal therapy (leuprolide acetate, medroxyprogesterone acetate, cyproterone acetate, flutamide, triptorelin) should be reserved for cases resistant to SSRIs and psychotherapy; for cases of recidivism; and for cases encompassing several paraphilias/paraphilic disorders, especially those causing more harm to others, e.g., sadistic disorder or pedophilic disorder. Combining various treatments seems prudent, though there is no evidence addressing treatment combinations. Treatment risks and side effects of all medications should always be discussed with the patient, even in cases of court-mandated treatment.

As Lussier and Piche ([5], p 158) wrote, "…an individual treated with androgen reduction therapy should have a baseline physical examination, laboratory assessment, including testosterone levels, and bone density evaluations, and these should be repeated every 6–12 months." They also advise a collaborative work of psychiatrist with an internist, family physician, or endocrinologist if androgen reducing therapy is used. Psychiatrists not comfortable using antiandrogens themselves or in collaboration with internists or endocrinologists should refer patients to specialists dealing with these disorders.

References

1. American Psychiatric Association. Diagnostic and statistical manual of mental disorders. 3rd ed. Washington, DC: American Psychiatric Association; 1980.
2. American Psychiatric Association. Diagnostic and statistical manual of mental disorders. 3rd ed., rev. Washington, DC: American Psychiatric Association; 1987.
3. American Psychiatric Association. Diagnostic and statistical manual of mental disorders. 5th ed. Arlington: American Psychiatric Association; 2013. p. 691–4.
4. Magnan V. Des exhibitionnistes. Les Archives Archives de l' Anthropologie Crimenelle et de Sciences Penales. 1890;5:456–71.
5. Lussier P, Piche L. Frotteurism: psychopathology and theory. In: Laws DR, O'Donohue WT, editors. Sexual deviance. Theory, assessment, and treatment. 2nd ed. New York: Guilford; 2008. p. 131–49.
6. von Kraft-Ebbing R. Psychopathia sexualis. The classic study of deviant sex. New York: Arcade; 2011.
7. Clark SK, Jeglic EL, Calkins C, Tatar JR. More than a nuisance: the prevalence and consequences of frotteurism and exhibitionism. Sex Abuse. 2016;28:3–19.
8. Krueger RB, Kaplan MS. Frotteurism: assessment and treatment. In: Laws DR, O'Donohue WT, editors. Sexual deviance. Theory, assessment, and treatment. 2nd ed. New York: Guilford; 2008. p. 150–63.
9. Harima K. Frotteurism (article in Japanese). Ryoikibetsu Shokogun Shirizu. 2003;39:294–6.
10. Horley J. Frotteurism: a term in search of an underlying disorder? J Sex Aggress. 2001;7:51–5.

11. Langstrom N. The DSM diagnostic criteria for exhibitionism, voyeurism, and frotteurism. Arch Sex Behav. 2010;39:317–24.
12. Johnson RS, Ostermeyer B, Sikes KA, Nelsen AJ, Coverdale JH. Prevalence and treatment of frotteurism in the community: a systematic review. J Am Acad Psychiatry Law. 2014;42:479–83.
13. Abel GG, Becker J, Mittelman M, Cunningham-Rathner J, Rouleau J, Murphy W. Self-reported sex crimes of nonincarcerated paraphiliacs. J Interpers Violence. 1987;2:3–25.
14. Becker JV, Stinson J, Tromp S, Messer G. Characteristics of individuals petitioned for civil commitment. Int J Offender Ther Comp Criminol. 2003;47:185–95.
15. Abel GG, Osborne C. The paraphilias. The extend and nature of sexually deviant and criminal behavior. Psychiatr Clin North Am. 1992;15:675–701.
16. Zolondek SC, Abel GG, Northey Jr WE, Jordan A. Self-reported behaviors of juvenile sexual offenders. J Interpers Violence. 2001;16:73–85.
17. Freund K, Watson R. Mapping the boundaries of courtship disorder. J Sex Res. 1990;27:589–606.
18. Freund K, Seto MC. Preferential rape in the theory of courtship disorder. Arch Sex Behav. 1998;27:433–43.
19. Cannas A, Solla P, Floris G, Tacconi P, Loi D, Marcia E, Marrosu MG. Hypersexual behavior, frotterurism and delusional jealousy in a young parkinsonian patients during dopaminergic therapy with pergolide: a rare case of iatrogenic paraphilia. Prog Neuropsychopharmacol Biol Psychiatry. 2006;30:1539–41.
20. Kuruvilla K, Joseph S. A case of frotteurism and its successful treatment by behavior therapy. Indian J Psychiatry. 1983;25:159–61.
21. Perilstein RD, Lipper S, Friendman LJ. Three cases if paraphilias responsive to fluoxetine treatment. J Clin Psychiatry. 1991; 52:169–70.
22. Patra AP, Bharadwaj B, Shaha KK, Das S, Raymane AP, Tripathi CS. Impulsive frotteurism. Med Sci Law. 2013;53:235–8.
23. Kalra G. The depressive façade in a case of compulsive sex behavior with frottage. Indian J Psychiatry. 2013;55:183–5.
24. Kruger RB, Kaplan MS. Depot-leuprolide acetate for treatment of paraphilias: a report of twelve cases. Arch Sex Behav. 2001;30:409–22.
25. Bradford JMW. The neurobiology, neuropharmacology, and pharmacological treatment of the paraphilias and compulsive sexual behavior. Can J Psychiatry. 2001;46:26–34.

Chapter 8
Sexual Masochism Disorder

Rebecca A. Wylie and Kevan R. Wylie

Introduction

Sexual masochism is listed as both an unconventional yet non-pathological sexual interest, i.e. a paraphilia, and a psychological disorder within the psychiatric diagnostic manual the DSM [1]. A paraphilia is defined as any 'intense and persistent' sexual interest that is atypical. This may include but is not limited to sexual arousal that is directed at non-human objects, children or non-consenting participants. Sexual masochism and the associated sexual masochism disorder specify recurrent and intense sexual fantasies, urges and behaviours arising from being humiliated, beaten, bound or otherwise made to suffer [1]. Reprinted with permission from the Diagnostic and Statistical Manual of Mental Disorders, Fifth edition, (Copyright 2013). American Psychiatric Association.

R.A. Wylie, B.Sc., M.Sc., M.B.Ps.S.
Fishawack Facilitate Limited, 28-30 Robert Street, Brighton, East Sussex BN1 4AH, UK
e-mail: rebecca.a.wylie@gmail.com

K.R. Wylie, M.D., F.R.C.P., F.R.C.Psych. (✉)
Department of Neurosciences, University of Sheffield, Western Bank, Sheffield, South Yorkshire S10 2TN, UK
e-mail: k.r.wylie@sheffield.ac.uk

R. Balon (ed.), *Practical Guide to Paraphilia and Paraphilic Disorders*, DOI 10.1007/978-3-319-42650-1_8

Masochism is categorised within the same subgroup as sexual sadism (*inflicting* humiliation, pain or suffering); as an algolagnic activity preference, i.e. that involving pain or suffering. (More information about sexual sadism is detailed in Chap. 9.)

The psychiatric literature has historically characterised paraphilic behaviours as disordered. Since first appearing within the DSM, paraphilias have been viewed as qualitatively different to mild engagement in sexual fantasy or role-play within adult sexuality [2]. However, there has been considerable debate about where to draw the line on what is considered normal and what is considered deviant, and therefore paraphilic. Changing perceived sexual norms according to culture and time make this even more difficult to define [3]. Many have argued that the inclusion of paraphilias within the DSM pathologises diverse sexual behaviours that should be considered as appearing along a spectrum of sexual behaviours [4].

The most recent edition of the DSM, DSM-5, is the first significant attempt to tackle this issue by distinguishing between paraphilic behaviours and paraphilic disorders. Therefore individuals may engage in some atypical sexual behaviour without being defined as having a mental disorder. Diagnosis of a paraphilic disorder is now made on the basis of distress and dysfunction [5]. It is thought that the revision for the ICD 11 will also reflect this differentiation [6].

This chapter will detail the diagnostic criteria of sexual masochism and associated disorder as well as a case example. The evidence surrounding the prevalence, psychopathology, possible aetiology and the functioning of individuals presenting with sexual masochism behaviours shall be discussed. Finally, clinical recommendations will be presented along with concluding comments.

Diagnostic Criteria

The criteria within the DSM-5 states that an individual with sexual masochism paraphilia will have experienced recurrent and intense sexual arousal that arises from fantasies, urges or behaviours of the act of being humiliated, bound or otherwise made to suffer, over a period of 6 months or more. To be diagnosed with sexual masochism disorder these fantasies, urges or behaviours must have caused significant clinical distress or impairment to an individual's daily functioning. The DSM-5 allows for further specifications within the diagnosis. Firstly, it is specified whether the individual also engages in sexual asphyxiation. This is the practice of achieving sexual arousal through restriction of breathing. Secondly, it is specified whether the individual is in a controlled environment, for example, in an institution where opportunities to practise masochistic activities are reduced. Thirdly, it is specified whether the individual is in full remission, this is where there has been no distress or impaired functioning over the last 5 years in an uncontrolled environment. The DSM-5 makes clear that the 6 month criteria is more of a guideline than strict rule, for example, a shorter period of time may still have a clear diagnosis. Reprinted with permission from the Diagnostic and Statistical Manual of Mental Disorders, Fifth edition, (Copyright 2013). American Psychiatric Association

The International Disease Classification of Mental and Behavioural disorders (ICD-10) defines sexual masochism as a preference for being the recipient of bondage, pain or humiliation [7]. The ICD-10 emphasises that a diagnosis of masochism should only be made when masochistic activity is the most important form of stimulation or is necessary for sexual gratification. Current proposals for changes to the revised ICD-11 suggest that the ICD will also aim to depathologise by distinguishing between paraphilic behaviours and disordered cases [6].

Case Example

The following case example details the notorious 'Spanner Trials' and is described in full in White [8]. The following case example has been chosen here as it examples a broad spectrum of sexual masochism activities as well as presenting key issues surrounding sexual masochism. Notably, these are issues of privacy, consent and perceptions.

In 1990, in the United Kingdom, a group of 16 gay men that had been engaging in consensual sadomasochistic activities were found guilty of assault and of aiding and abetting assault. Photographs and video footage of the sexual activities intended for private use by the involved participants were seized by the Police and used in Court as evidence to charge the men. The videotapes were reported to document a vast array of sadomasochistic behaviours including but not limited to 'beatings of the buttocks, legs, cock and balls with leather straps, canes, nettles etc. Hot wax being dripped onto genitals, torsos, legs etc. Play piercings of tits, scrotums, cock knobs, shafts and foreskins. Genital application of heat (hair driers) and cold (ice cubes). Genital bondage and manipulation etc., ball weights, safe electrical play…Scrotal stretching and pinning out with needles etc. Nipple and cock branding' (p 169) [8].

The men were convicted after being denied a defence that the activity was consensual. The Judge refused this plea on the basis that the court must distinguish between what is acceptable within a civilised society and what is not, deciding that sadomasochistic activities fell into the latter category. Furthermore, the Court of Appeal deemed that it was not 'in the public interest' to allow individuals to be engaging in sadomasochistic activities.

Following this ruling, several of the convicted men appealed to the European Court of Human Rights on the grounds that the UK Government had violated their right to privacy. However the convictions remained as it was concluded that the government has a right to intervene if this is in the interest of public health.

The evidence used in court was heavily criticised as footage had been excessively edited with the effect of portraying an inaccurate and incomplete picture of the activities. It was argued that the editing process had removed all context of the activities including consent and evidence of pleasure. The Lords involved in the hearing described the activities as 'a cult of violence' and stated that 'pleasure derived from the infliction of pain is an evil thing.'

It is clear from these comments and from the entire handling of this case that there were significant misunderstandings of sadomasochistic activities and negative perceptions held. This resulted in the sadomasochistic behaviours being deemed to be barbaric, dangerous and abusive. The impression from this case is of the horror with which wider society viewed these diverse behaviours and society's desire to police and correct these.

It has been argued that this criminalisation of sadomasochism has led to sadomasochistic practices now being less safe for practitioners as it discourages individuals from freely engaging in and discussing such activities [8]. This has resulted in individuals being less able to access safe sex literature and social networks to share safety advice. In addition, White cites a case whereby an individual engaged in breath restriction on his own for fear of involving his partner and died as a result.

Summary of evidence

Prevalence

The true prevalence of sexual masochism disorder is unknown. An Australian study that conducted telephone interviews on over 19,000 respondents found that approximately 2.2 % of males and 1.3 % of females had been involved in bondage and discipline, sadomasochism or dominance and submission in the last 12 months [9]. However, due to the private and personal nature of this topic it is unlikely that a telephone survey will reveal true prevalence rates. Indeed, a recent comparison of survey methods found that an Internet survey produced significantly higher rates of acknowledgement of paraphilic experiences than a comparable telephone survey [10]. Furthermore this gives no indication as to the prevalence of disordered cases, or masochistic activities in particular.

Connolly [11] found that only 0.8 % of self-identified BDSM practitioners reported feeling frequently distressed by their involvement in BDSM. The prevalence of disordered cases may be particularly difficult to ascertain due to frequent changes in the criterion for a clinical diagnosis [3].

Numerous studies have indicated that the prevalence of masochistic fantasies is high. For example, Joyal, Cossette and Lapiierre [12] surveyed 1516 individuals recruited in Quebec on their sexual fantasies. The themes of domination and submission in fantasies were specifically explored and it was found that 30–60 % of the women surveyed reported sexual fantasies of being tied up, being dominated, being spanked or whipped and being forced to have sex. Men also reported similar fantasies, though to a lesser degree. Critelli and Bivona [13] conducted a review of the literature and report a similar finding, with 9–17 % of respondents indicating that erotic rape fantasies were frequent or preferred fantasies, these may be explained by masochism. It is unknown what the level of behavioural engagement was in these cases. However, surveys have also noted that individuals with paraphilic interests do not experience these only in terms of fantasies but also as desires to experience these [10]. This evidence suggests that masochistic fantasies at the least are commonplace. Joyal and Carpentier [10] found interests in masochism to be at a level above that considered statistically unusual. Some have argued that this indicates that masochism should be considered along a spectrum of normal sexuality [4].

Variability

It is important to note that the motivations and meanings behind masochistic behaviours frequently vary between individuals. For example, some individuals might be seeking the psychological effects of engaging in masochistic behaviours whilst for others the sensory experience may be more important [14]. Some individuals may engage in these activities for the challenge, the experience of pain or the close connection that they may feel with their partner during this shared experience. Likewise, individuals may have different patterns of sexual behaviours according to the different effects these have. Sandnabba et al. [15] conducted a smallest space analysis on data from 184 sadomasochistically orientated individuals and found evidence of four qualitatively different facets of sexual behaviour; administration of pain, humiliation, physical restriction and hypermasculinity.

The practice of masochistic behaviours falls in with a catalogue of other diverse sexual behaviours that are collectively known as BDSM. This acronym has developed to refer to Bondage and Domination, Dominance/Submission and Sadomasochism and/or slave/Master interactions [16]. The BDSM community consists of a wide cross section of ethnicities, ages, occupations, genders and sexual identities and members of the BDSM community frequently positively identify as such [11].

Individuals may solely practise masochistic behaviours or they may also engage in sadistic behaviours. Sandnabba et al. [15] found that 22.7 % of their respondents identified as both sadistic and masochistic, 27 % identified as mainly sadistic and 50.2 % identified as mainly masochistic.

Psychopathology

There has been remarkable debate over the inclusion of the paraphilias within the psychiatric diagnostic manuals. Many have argued that practitioners of paraphilic behaviours do not fit the criteria of mental disorders and that their inclusion pathologises groups of individuals that engage in unconventional sexual practices [17]. Studies have found practitioners of masochism to be no more prone to psychological distress or mental instability than other groups. In fact, this group reported higher levels of employment as compared to a sub-group of practitioners of sadism and the non-sadomasochistic community [18]. This has led some to question why paraphilias are even still listed within the DSM, especially since it is acknowledged that the behaviours are not causing problems [5].

It has been observed that there can be psychological benefits from engaging in BDSM activities including heightened meaning making [16]. Krueger [19] reports that sadomasochistic activities might be associated with reduced stress and that it increases relationship closeness.

The ICD-10 specifies that a diagnosis of sexual masochism is dependent upon the individual viewing masochistic activity as the most important sexual activity, or necessary for sexual gratification. It has been shown that individuals with a preference for sexual masochism demonstrate genital and subjective sexual arousal to both masochistic and conventional sex stimuli, i.e. it is non-specific [20]. This evidence supports the notion that the practice of masochism itself is not necessarily disordered but is a preference since masochistic activity is not essential for arousal. It is noted that this sample did not specifically include individuals identifying as strongly masochistic. However these findings point towards a broadening of sexual preference rather than a narrowing of interest.

On the other hand, there is also evidence to include sexual masochism and sexual masochism disorder within our classifications. There is wide recognition that masochistic behaviours carry significant risk, and have in some cases been reported to result in severe injury or death. This is particularly true during the practice of restricting breathing to produce sexual arousal. Krueger [19] reports on a study that found sexual asphyxiation to be responsible for 50 fatalities in the United States yearly and many individuals have reported masochistic fantasies during this practice. It is argued that this warrants the continued inclusion within the DSM and stated that for cases where behaviour is out of control the diagnostic criteria is suitable to capture this [19].

Alternative definitions of paraphilias have been proposed to address these issues. For example, Federoff [5] suggested that paraphilias should instead be defined as 'a persistent or recurrent sexual interest that involves non-consent or interferes with sexual function.' This is in line with attitudes moving away from pathologising non-reproductive sexual activities to those that pathologise non-consent in sexual interactions [21].

Clinical Samples

It could be argued that it is not surprising that studies using community samples do not find psychopathology since this is exactly what the latest revision of the DSM expresses. Of interest though is whether individuals with sexual masochism disorder, i.e. clinical samples, demonstrate pathology.

A recent exploratory study specifically sampled patients that were seeking treatment for problematic sexual behaviour or sexual addiction. Hopkins et al. [4] investigated the associations between personality, psychopathology and engagement in sadomasochistic behaviours using the Minnesota Multiphasic Inventory-2 along with measures of sexual thoughts and behaviours in 980 patients. The authors categorised participants based on whether they were high or low risk. Individuals that were low risk sought out humiliation and loss of power whereas those that were considered high risk engaged in sexual asphyxiation. Within the sample it was found that several forms of psychopathology and psychological disturbance were predictive of engagement in sadomasochistic behaviours. It was observed that the predictors varied by gender and by the level of risk. Some of these predictors included feelings of worthlessness, guilt and antisocial behaviours in women and schizotypal characteristics, hypomanic activation and anxiety in men. Limitation to this study is that there was no differentiation between the individuals that were practising sadistic behaviours and those practising masochistic behaviours. Nonetheless these result show support for the recent amendments to the DSM in that it is the individuals that are distressed or experiencing dysfunction due to their paraphilic behaviour that are likely to show pathology.

Etiological Theories

There are numerous theories surrounding masochism and sadism. More traditionally the development of sadomasochistic behaviours has been viewed in terms of individual pathology, symptoms and maladjustment [18]. It has frequently been theorised that the development of sadomasochistic interests is dependent upon childhood experiences, particularly the experiences of childhood trauma or abuse. It is also theorised that masochistic activities are indicative of sexual deficiency in adulthood [15].

There has been little empirical evidence to support any of these perspectives. Powls and Davies [17] conducted a review and concluded that the majority of individuals practising sadomasochistic behaviours did not suffer from childhood abuse. Telephone interviews with over 10,000 men and 9000 women across Australia revealed that individuals who had engaged in BDSM in the past year were not more likely to have ever been sexually coerced [22]. Furthermore this survey found no association with any of the sexual difficulties in adulthood asked about in the survey.

However, it is of note that Hopkins et al. [4] found some evidence of higher rates of abuse within their clinical sample. Furthermore, Nordling et al. [23] found that the small proportion of respondents that did report childhood sexual abuse were also more likely to have attempted suicide, show poorer social adjustment and to have sought psychological support. This again supports the recommendations to clearly distinguish between behaviour and disorder.

Other perspectives take a social and cultural stance, recognising that individuals are influenced by their social context. For example, Weinberg [24] explained sadomasochistic behaviours as being based on socialisation and a gradual understanding and reinforcement of the norms and values of the sadomasochistic community. This is supported by evidence that the onset of tendencies is late and gradual [5]. Sandnabba et al. [15] found that respondents whom were sadomasochistically orientated reported a median age of between 18 and 20 years old for first awareness of sadomasochistic interest.

Some have suggested that paraphilias emerge as a way of coping with or protecting against internal emotions such as anxiety [25]. These emotions may arise from problems occurring during childhood such as abuse, thus explaining any associations. This process can be viewed of as cyclical whereby the individual uses fantasies as a temporary escape from feelings of distress. Gradually these fantasies may become behaviours that produce sexual arousal and later lead to feelings of shame before the individual may begin the cycle again. Breaking this cycle may be a clinical aim.

A Negative Label

It has been argued that research used to inform the DSM has relied heavily on both clinical and forensic samples. Importantly, this fails to distinguish between coercive behaviours and the consensual behaviours that are integral to BDSM practices [16]. This can result in the BDSM community being unfairly represented and stigmatised. Forensic samples are frequently used despite little evidence to suggest that masochism leads to criminality [19]. The effects of such negative associations may be clinically significant. Kolmes et al. [26] reported evidence of Health Professionals demonstrating biased, inadequate and inappropriate care, mistaking sadomasochistic behaviours as abuse. Patients report that clinicians fail to understand their relationships and instead label their activities as pathological [14]. This is also a problem for individuals outside of clinical environments. Traditional views that paraphilic behaviours equate to mental illness can have negative psychological impacts on individuals [17]. Further, despite recent advances in distinguishing between paraphilias and paraphilic disorders, it is noted that many individuals still see these as the same [5].

Negative labels held by society have been argued to make it difficult for individuals in abusive relationships disguised as BDSM interactions to seek and receive support from clinicians, police and peers [27]. Pitagora [27] interviewed four individuals that had experienced abuse in the context of what they thought was BDSM with their partner. These individuals experienced non-consensual violence that was not in line with healthy and consensual dominance/submission. Pitagora expressed that society's lack of understanding is likely to have contributed to some individuals not seeking support.

Treatment Options

Not all sexually masochistic behaviour is clinically significant. Treatment should only be for patients who are experiencing distress or dysfunction, or those that are at risk of putting themselves in danger [3]. There is minimal research that investigates treatment options for non-criminal paraphilias. Therapy of various forms (analytical, behavioural or cognitive) may include exploring themes of submission in sexual power (imbalance) dynamics, childhood sexuality, guilt, shame, humiliation, punishment and pain. For some, the pain avoids any emotional distress. Consideration of the constructed role-play scenes and use, or lack of use, of contracts, e.g. safe words can also be helpful. There may be comorbidities to manage such as anxiety, social role and self-esteem issues.

Recommendations

In line with the recent revisions to the DSM and with the latest research on sexual masochism it is recommended that any necessary clinical interventions aim to empower individuals. The emphasis should be on changing perceptions rather than behaviour per se and enabling individuals to take control of their own sexual expression. It is acknowledged that pharmacological treatments may be necessary to reduce sexual fantasies or behaviour when an individual continues to experience distress from their masochism or when they put themselves at risk of harm, e.g. asphyxiation, bodily injury or blood loss. No medications are specifically licenced for sexual masochism disorder but SSRI medications may decrease the preoccupation and sexual urges and behaviours and may be best suited for those individuals who have comorbid anxiety, depression or obsessive compulsive disorders. This treatment option should be in partnership with the patient understanding the reality and extent of the danger posed from these behaviours.

A structured therapeutic environment is recommended to facilitate difficult conversations surrounding this private and personal experience. There may be a need for the clinician to lead therapeutic conversations in order to ensure coverage of essential but sensitive topics, for example, checking that individuals are not being exploited or experiencing abuse.

Given the potentially serious consequences associated with sadomasochistic activities, it has previously been recommended, and is here too, that clinicians assess for sexual addiction and high-risk behaviours whilst working with patients seeking treatment for such behaviours [13]. It has been found that patients with paraphilic interests that also suffer from hyper sexuality are significantly more likely to report a history of criminality and of substance abuse than patients with hyper sexuality but no paraphilic interests [28]. This group were also more likely to report novelty seeking as the symptom of or motivator of their sexual problems. Therefore these may necessitate different treatment options.

Different motivations and goals may have different therapeutic implications [29]. For example, if the goal of masochistic activities is to self-punish due to underlying feelings of guilt then this is fundamentally different to any noxious consequences of behaviour intended solely to produce a sexual arousal from the experience of pain itself.

It is important to note that not all patients will necessarily present with issues surrounding their sexual behaviour. Rather, any paraphilic behaviours will emerge as areas of functioning are explored (Curen, 2016, personal correspondence). At this point a patient may accept this association, or dropout of treatment if they believe this association has been misjudged. Crucially, not all patients will want to abandon these behaviours and should not be expected to, for many individuals being part of the BDSM scene is a positive aspect of their lives, and their paraphilia does not cause distress or harm.

The traditional and prevailing associations between paraphilias and mental illness may mean that patients approach clinicians with concern that their behaviour is pathological [5]. It is crucially important to diagnose only when diagnostic criteria is firmly met due to the negative psychological impact this could have on an individual.

Clinicians' personal opinions are particularly important if they are misinformed about practices and thus hold negative judgements and biases [5]. Therefore, education about practices is essential, as is recognition of when a patient's behaviour is disordered and treatment is needed.

Conclusion

Sexual masochism is an unconventional sexual interest whereby individuals experience arousal relating to fantasies, urges or behaviours of the act of being humiliated, bound or otherwise made to suffer. The psychiatric literature has traditionally viewed this behaviour as disordered. However there is little evidence to suggest that individuals practising sexual masochism experience any kinds of psychopathology, and it has strongly been argued that the distinction between normal and abnormal sexual behaviour is arbitrary and inappropriately pathologises behaviours that should be considered along a normal spectrum of behaviour. The DSM-5 is the first attempt to address these issues, clearly distinguishing between behaviour and disorder.

Evidence of the prevailing negative views surrounding sexual masochism and the effects these can have on individuals indicates a need to educate both clinicians and the wider society in order to demystify this atypical behaviour and begin to eliminate prejudice, ensure safe practice and reduce distress.

However, it is also necessary to recognise that this behaviour can become clinically significant and for health professionals to understand treatment routes in these instances. There is evidence to suggest that some etiological theories may be relevant in cases where sexual masochism behaviour is disordered, and this may inform treatment options. When embarking on a clinical route it is particularly important that there is shared decision-making in treatment options due to the sensitive, personal and subjective issues surrounding masochism.

References

1. American Psychiatric Association. Diagnostic and statistical manual of mental disorders. 5th ed. Arlington: American Psychiatric Association; 2013.
2. First MB. DSM-5 and paraphilic disorders. J Am Acad Psychiatry Law. 2014;42(2):191–201.
3. McManus MA, Hargreaves P, Rainbow L, Alison LJ. Paraphilias: definition, diagnosis and treatment. F1000prime Rep. 2013;5:36.
4. Hopkins TA, Brawner CA, Meyer M, Zawilinski L, Carnes PJ, Green BA. MMPI-2 correlates of sadomasochism in a sexual addiction sample: contrasting and men and women. Sex Addict Compulsivity. 2016;23(1):114–40.
5. Fedoroff JP. Forensic and diagnostic concerns arising from the proposed DSM-5 criteria for sexual paraphilic disorder. J Am Acad Psychiatry Law. 2011;39(2):238–41.
6. Wylie KR. Paraphilia behaviour and disorders. In: Wylie KR, editor. ABC of sexual health. 3rd ed. London: Wiley; 2015. p. 90–2.
7. World Health Organization. The ICD-10 classification of mental and behavioural disorders: clinical descriptions and diagnostic guidelines. Geneva: World Health Organization; 1992.
8. White C. The Spanner trials and the changing law on sadomasochism in the UK. J Homosex. 2006;50(2–3):167–87.
9. Richters J, Grulich AE, Visser RO, Smith A, Rissel CE. Sex in Australia: autoerotic, esoteric and other sexual practices engaged in by a representative sample of adults. Aust N Z J Public Health. 2003;27(2):180–90.
10. Joyal CC, Carpentier J. The prevalence of paraphilic interests and behaviors in the general population: a provincial survey. J Sex Res. 2016:1–11.
11. Connolly PH. Psychological functioning of bondage/domination/sado-masochism (BDSM) practitioners. J Psychol Human Sex. 2006;18(1):79–120.
12. Joyal CC, Cossette A, Lapierre V. What exactly is an unusual sexual fantasy? J Sex Med. 2015;12(2):328–40.
13. Critelli JW, Bivona JM. Women's erotic rape fantasies: an evaluation of theory and research. J Sex Res. 2008;45(1):57–70.
14. Williams DJ. Different (Painful¡) strokes for different folks: a general overview of sexual sadomasochism (SM) and its diversity. Sex Addict Compulsivity. 2006;13(4):333–46.
15. Sandnabba NK, Santtila P, Alison L, Nordling N. Demographics, sexual behaviour, family background and abuse experiences of

practitioners of sadomasochistic sex: a review of recent research. Sex Relation Ther. 2002;17(1):39–55.
16. Pitagora D. Consent vs. coercion: BDSM interactions highlight a fine but immutable line. New School Psychol Bull. 2013;10(1):27–36.
17. Powls J, Davies J. A descriptive review of research relating to sadomasochism: considerations for clinical practice. Deviant Behav. 2012;33(3):223–34.
18. Cross PA, Matheson K. Understanding sadomasochism: an empirical examination of four perspectives. J Homosex. 2006;50(2–3):133–66.
19. Krueger RB. The DSM diagnostic criteria for sexual masochism. Arch Sex Behav. 2010;39(2):346–56.
20. Chivers ML, Roy C, Grimbos T, Cantor JM, Seto MC. Specificity of sexual arousal for sexual activities in men and women with conventional and masochistic sexual interests. Arch Sex Behav. 2014;43(5):931–40.
21. Giami A. Between DSM and ICD: paraphilias and the transformation of sexual norms. Arch Sex Behav. 2015;44(5):1127–38.
22. Richters J, De Visser RO, Rissel CE, Grulich AE, Smith A. Demographic and psychosocial features of participants in bondage and discipline, "sadomasochism" or dominance and submission (BDSM): data from a national survey. J Sex Med. 2008;5(7):1660–8.
23. Nordling N, Sandnabba NK, Santtila P. The prevalence and effects of self-reported childhood sexual abuse among sadomasochistically oriented males and females. J Child Sex Abus. 2000;9(1):53–63.
24. Weinberg TS. Sadomasochism in the United States: a review of recent sociological literature. J Sex Res. 1987;23(1):50–69.
25. Baumeister RF. Masochism as escape from self. J Sex Res. 1988;25(1):28–59.
26. Kolmes K, Stock W, Moser C. Investigating bias in psychotherapy with BDSM clients. J Homosex. 2006;50(2–3):301–24.
27. Pitagora D. Intimate partner violence in sadomasochistic relationships. Sex Relation Ther. 2016;31(1):95–108.
28. Sutton KS, Stratton N, Pytyck J, Kolla NJ, Cantor JM. Patient characteristics by type of hypersexuality referral: a quantitative chart review of 115 consecutive male cases. J Sex Marital Ther. 2015;41(6):563–80.
29. Kernberg OF. Clinical constellations of masochistic psychopathology. In: Holtzman D, Kulish N, editors. The clinical problem of masochism. Lanham: Jason Aronson; 2012. p. 15–27.

Chapter 9
Sexual Sadism Disorder

David V. Hamilton and Jordan Rosen

Introduction

Sexual sadism disorder is a condition associated with sexual arousal resulting from the suffering of another person. Formulating a precise definition of the disorder has proved challenging through the years on a number of fronts: not being overly inclusive so as to pathologize or stigmatize consensual sexual activity, yet constructing diagnostic criteria that are sensitive enough to allow for study and treatment in both forensic and non-forensic populations. Sexual Sadism has been difficult to identify, and has challenges associated in treating it through both pharmacologic and psychotherapeutic avenues. Studies have noted that the diagnosis has serious and long-term consequences for the patient [1], so it is important to draw a distinction between pathology and variants of normal sexual behavior. How the disorder is defined also has a large role in how we identify the disorder; the definition should provide clinical utility in linking the disorder

D.V. Hamilton, M.D., M.A. (✉) • J. Rosen, M.D.
Department of Psychiatry and Neurobehavioral Sciences, University of Virginia, 1215 Lee Street, Charlottesville, VA 22903, USA
e-mail: dvh2g@virginia.edu

R. Balon (ed.), *Practical Guide to Paraphilia and Paraphilic Disorders*, DOI 10.1007/978-3-319-42650-1_9

with people who are prone to sexual offending and recidivism [2]. Much of the literature on the subject is in forensic populations alone. There is a paucity of research outside of the forensic population. Moreover, there is scant research on treatments, either pharmacologic or psychotherapeutic, specifically with regard to sexual sadism. However, given the damages the disorder can cause when a patient does offend, intervention is mandated. As we shall demonstrate, the available treatment modalities are limited and have been largely appropriated from the extant research on the treatment of paraphilias in general.

Diagnosis

The standard diagnostic criteria as stated in the ICD-10 (International Classification of Diseases, 10th Revision) [3] and DSM-5 (Diagnostic and Statistical Manual of Mental Disorders, 5th Edition) [4] are as follows:

ICD

In the International Statistical Classification of Diseases and Related Health Problems sexual sadism is conceptualized as a paraphilia with "A disorder characterized by recurrent sexual urges, fantasies, or behaviors involving acts (real, not simulated) in which the psychological or physical suffering of a victim is sexually exciting to the individual" [3]. Of note, depending on how one parses the parenthetic "real, not simulated," the criterion that there must be a lack of consent does not appear in the ICD definition of sexual sadism, which would seem to identify some practitioners of BDSM (i.e., Bondage Discipline Dominance Submission Sadism Masochism) as diagnosable sexual sadists. As we shall see, the evolution of the DSM criteria though its multiple editions has made the lack of consent of particular importance to the application of the diagnosis.

DSM

While the DSM-III established the core of what the disorder would become in its current iteration, the DSM diagnosis has evolved through the 4th edition, 4th edition Text Revision (DSM 4-TR), as well as the 5th edition. Notably, the A criterion of the DSM-III included sexual urges and sexually arousing fantasies, which was broadened to include behaviors as well in later additions. Additionally, the B criterion has evolved as well. In DSM-III, the criterion included acting on or being markedly distressed by urges. However in DSM-IV having acting on the urges was removed, but impairment in social, occupational, or other areas of important functioning was added. The DSM-IV-TR saw the restoration of having acted on the urges, but added to this having acted on these urges with nonconsenting persons, thereby not pathologizing consensual BDSM activity [5–7]. A comparison of the previous editions is noted in Table 9.1.

In DSM-5, sexual sadism disorder is defined as "recurrent and intense sexual arousal from the physical or psychological suffering of another person, as manifested by fantasies, urges, or behaviors."

Symptom criteria for sexual sadism disorder in DSM-5 (Reprinted with the permission from the Diagnostic and Statistical Manual of Mental Disorders, Fifth Edition, (Copyright 2013). American Psychiatric Association) are as follows:

A. *Over a period of at least 6 months, recurrent and intense sexual arousal from the physical or psychological suffering of another person, as manifested by fantasies, urges, or behaviors.*
B. *The individual has acted on these sexual urges with a nonconsenting person, or the sexual urges and fantasies cause clinically significant distress or impairment in social, occupational, or other important areas of functioning.*

Two specifiers are also added: "In a controlled environment" where opportunities to engage in the behaviors are restricted, and "In full remission" when criterion B has not been met for at least 5 years in an uncontrolled environment [4].

Table 9.1 Changes in the DSM Criteria across editions [4–6] (Reprinted with permission from the Diagnostic and Statistical Manual of Mental Disorders, Fifth Edition, (Copyright 2013). American Psychiatric Association)

DSM-IIIR	DSM-IV	DSM-IVR
A. Over a period of at least 6 months, recurrent intense sexual urges and sexually arousing fantasies involving acts (real, not simulated) in which the psychological or physical suffering (including humiliation) of the victim is sexually exciting to the person	A. Over a period of at least 6 months, recurrent, intense sexually arousing fantasies, sexual urges, or behaviors involving acts (real, not simulated) in which the psychological or physical suffering (including humiliation) of the victim is sexually exciting to the person	A. Over a period of at least 6 months, recurrent, intense sexually arousing fantasies, sexual urges, or behaviors involving acts (real, not simulated) in which the psychological or physical suffering (including humiliation) of the victim is sexually exciting to the person
B. The person has acted on these urges or is markedly distressed by them	B. The fantasies, sexual urges, or behaviors cause clinically significant distress or impairment in social, occupational, or other important areas of functioning	B. The person has acted on these urges with a nonconsenting person, or the sexual urges or behaviors cause marked distress or interpersonal difficulty

A careful defining of this order is necessary to differentiate sexual sadism from consensual BDSM activities. The DSM-5 emphasizes in the B criterion that the patient has acted on their desires with a nonconsenting person. The ICD-10 is not as explicit, though it also offers a qualifier that may aid in this differentiation by stating that the preoccupation must be with acts that are "real, not simulated" [3]. However, the ICD-10 phraseology would still diagnose as sexual sadist those BDSM practitioners who inflict real pain with a consenting partner. Whether the application of the diagnosis is warranted in this population, and by what rubric one would decide whether it is warranted, is beyond the scope of this manual.

A careful history should be taken including focus on development and content of sexual fantasies, sexual experiences or assaults throughout the patient's life, frequency and masturbation practice, detailed exploration of both sadistic and other paraphilic fantasies, pornography consumption, behaviors and fantasies within and beyond relationships including with prostitutes, and previous criminal acts and prosecutions.

Although many researchers conclude that the sexual arousal in the disorder comes from violent or humiliating behavior [8–11], some believe that it's more based in the victim's response to the violence or humiliation or due to a feeling of power and control obtained from inflicting these behaviors on others [12]. Yet others contend that the arousal is actually generated from the pain and fear the victim incurs [1, 13].

Due to the high risk for sexual offense recidivism [14, 15], as well as the burden that pharmacotherapy imposes, it is important to be both sensitive and specific with diagnosis of this disorder. Often, practitioners have to rely on patients' self-reports of their fantasies and acts, especially when the patient has either not offended or been caught offending yet. This poses a significant problem as many patients may be unwilling or unlikely to report such fantasies given concerns for legal or social consequences.

Beyond subjective report, there are both direct and indirect measures of preference for sexual violence (PSV). The most direct measure is phallometric assessment (i.e., penile plethysmography), which is a method of measuring sexual arousal via changes in penile tumescence while the patient is presented with various sexual events that have a number of variables including degree of consent, coercion, and violence [16]. Phallometric assessment is a method that has not consistently identified sexual sadists from nonsexual sadist in rapist populations, though this could be due to poor validity of the DSM diagnosis [17]. Indirect measures of PSV include such psychometric techniques as the Implicit Association Test to reveal beliefs or attitudes that subjects may be unwilling or unable to report, or measuring of Viewing Time, which records the length of time spent viewing an image of sexual interest passively while a subject is asked to apply a Likert scale to indicate interest in the image. Larue et al. demonstrated that both of these indirect measures were able to predict PSV [18].

Crime scene behaviors can have high reliability and validity for making a diagnosis of sexual sadism [19]. The Severe Sexual Sadism Scale (SSSS) is an 11-item, yes/no screening tool that delineates behavioral indicators of sexual sadism within forensic cases that could be sexual in nature [20, 21].

With regard to predicting violent recidivism, the Sex Offender Risk Appraisal Guide (SORAG), a modification of the violence appraisal guide by adding items that dealt with sexual offenses, as well as penile plethysmography, have outperformed the DSM [22]. The SORAG is a 14 item inventory 14 items assess child and adolescent adjustment, criminal history, psychopathy, and atypical sexual interests: living with both biological parents until age 16, elementary school maladjustment, history of alcohol problems, marital history, nonviolent offense history, victim sex/age, failure on prior conditional release, age at index offense, meeting DSM criteria for any personality disorder and for schizophrenia, phallometrically measured atypical sexual arousal, and Psychopathy Checklist-Revised score [23, 24].

Prevalence

For the same reasons that diagnosis by history taking along is problematic in this disorder, prevalence is difficult to ascertain. Within forensic samples, a range of prevalence from 2 to 30 % has been reported [25], and in samples from incarcerated sexual offenders from Austria, a DSM-IV diagnosis of sexual sadism was present in 6 % and was as high as 10 % amongst rapists [26]. Recent taxometric analyses utilizing the SSSS suggested that forensic sexual sadism may be better described in a dimensional rather than a categorical manner [27]. Little data has been collected on the prevalence of sexual sadism outside of the forensic population. Sexual sadism is predominantly found in males and usually has an onset that parallels puberty.

Clinical Example

Note: The following is a fictionalized account of a patient with SSD presenting for treatment outside of a forensic context. Though the prevalence of SSD would suggest otherwise, the stigma and potential for legal consequences make the non-forensic presentation a rare event, thus necessitating the generation of a fictional patient.

Mr. D, a 29-year-old garbage disposal repairman, with no previous psychiatric history, presented to the outpatient psychiatric clinic on referral from his primary care physician following what the patient described as a "relapse" to his addiction to pornography. When asked about the details of his "pornography addiction," the patient demonstrated obvious signs of distress, appearing anxious, and was initially guarded about the nature of the pornography consumed. A psychiatric interview revealed some neurovegetative symptoms of depression, including difficulty initiating and maintaining sleep, feelings of decreased self-esteem, guilt regarding his fixation on sex, and anhedonia. He denied problems with energy, concentration, or thoughts of suicide. He denied any current or past symptoms of mania or hypomania, symptoms of psychosis, including perceptual disturbances, delusions, or negative symptoms of psychosis. While he denied any compulsive behaviors, he reports ego-dystonic obsessive thoughts regarding his sexual fantasies that were intrusive to the point of impacting his ability to concentrate on other subjects. Finally, he denied any past or current use of substances, stating that he has 2–3 drinks every other month, typically during the holidays or some other special occasion.

On interview, the patient presented as an attractive, well-developed, well-nourished male of European descent who was well dressed and appeared to have intact hygiene. He displayed normal eye contact (though averted when describing the content of his sexual fantasies and behaviors), speech patterns, and a logical, linear thought process. The patient described having an unremarkable childhood with an intact family, to whom he showed neither abnormal amounts of hostility nor pathological attachment to either his father, who also worked as a garbage disposal repairman, or his mother, who was primarily a homemaker though also worked part-time outside the home as a cashier. He described himself as a “late bloomer,” entering puberty early in the sophomore year of high school. Within his peer group, the sharing of illicitly obtained pornographic material was the primary activity that signified membership within the group. From his first exposure to hard core pornography around age 13, Mr. D found himself drawn to images in which the male was overtly dominating the woman, and soon discovered the BDSM subculture. He developed the persona of the outsider due to an inability to bond with his peers over conventionally arousing pornographic material, though at the time his experienced this as being “edgier” than his peers.

The patient recounted taking seasonal jobs in his largely agricultural community. During the Halloween season, he worked as a haunted house employee, draping his costume creatively to conceal his arousal from both the clients and his coworkers. Between shifts, he would slip away to masturbate to the memory of the screams and expressions of terror on the girls’ and women’s faces. One autumn, when the patient was a 22-year-old college senior, he was reported for rubbing his genitals during a haunted house performance, an incident he called an embarrassing “slip.” He was dismissed from his position but no charges were filed and his university was not informed. While he has not suffered legal consequences from his sexual fixation, he states that he has suffered several consequences. He has never had a significant romantic relationship because, he states, "how could I love a person and only feel pleasure from their suffering?" He also has no close non-romantic relationships, fearing that he would be "outted" and seen as a "pervert."

Mr. D was adamant that he has never victimized anyone. He reported that he has had consensual sex with a few women. While he has been able to remain tumescent and, on two occasions, achieve orgasm he finds that the momentary pleasure he experience from libidinous discharge is soon replaced by feelings of guilt and anger that he cannot achieve "real sexual fulfillment." He claimed to have attempted to hire a prostitute whom he could torture, but this encounter proved unsatisfactory when he crossed her boundary regarding pain tolerance and she summoned her pimp. They then stole his wallet, watch, and tie clip in addition to the cash already dispensed for the prostitute's services. In addition to these negative outcomes, he came to understand that the crossing of boundaries was what he found so sexually fulfilling.

Upon understanding that his primary arousal pattern was the nonconsensual infliction of sexual violence, he began to find himself able to think of little else, having difficulty achieving sleep, and unable to enjoy anything other than "rape scenes," pornographic material in which the woman is, real or simulated, depicted as being violently raped. The patient was started on fluoxetine 10 mg po qDay, with a plan to increase to 20 mg qDay in 1 week. He was also encouraged to begin a log of his sexual activity, including estimated time spent in sexual fantasizing, masturbatory activity, and sexual activity with a partner. Finally, the boundaries regarding the limitations of the doctor–patient relationship were explained; for instance, he was told that any specific plans to commit a crime would need to be reported to the authorities. He seemed to be familiar with these relatively subtle aspects of the doctor–patient privilege.

Since the patient is seeking help outside of a forensic context, it is difficult to gauge the level of honesty with which he conveys his struggles. Given his relative youth, access to online resources, and at least a passing familiarity with the legality of confidentiality rights, it is possible that the patient is concealing a history of acting on his sexually sadistic impulses. In spite of this uncertainty, his clear eagerness to suppress and change the sexual preferences that have long kept him socially isolated is encouraging.

Recommendations

The primary goals of treatment, as in any paraphilic disorder, are to control sexually sadistic fantasies and behaviors and decrease the level of distress associated with their urges and fantasies. It should be emphasized that there are very little data on SSD in general, and still fewer data on the treatment of SSD in the non-forensic population. While both psychotherapeutic and pharmacologic treatments are important in the treatment of sexual sadism, pharmacologic intervention should be first line in severe cases where victimization is a higher risk [28]. In these cases, treatment should still be augmented with psychotherapy, especially behavioral therapy [29, 30]. It is important to note that all the information below is related to studies on paraphilias in general, and not specifically patients with sexual sadism disorder (again, given the paucity of data on SSD and specifically SSD in the non-forensic population). Further, most studies have been performed on male patients with little data on female patients with paraphilic disorders.

There are three main classes of medication that are used for the treatment of this disorder: SSRIs, antiandrogens, GNRH analogues, with the latter having the most promise in terms of its effects on recidivism and side effect tolerability. A high standard of informed consent is necessary when dealing with hormonal agents, with careful explanation of the likely side effects, both sexual and otherwise [31]. In sexual sadism disorder, the patient often is offered therapy under some degree of coercion, though this type of action should be taken by a court or other competent body and should not specify the actual treatment to be used but instead force the patient to comply with a medication regimen that is negotiated with a practitioner with the required experience and training to prescribe such a treatment [28]. Regardless of the method by which a patient comes to receive pharmacotherapy, due to both intended and side effects of medication, compliance is often low especially when depot preparations are not used.

While there are only limited case reports of the use of SSRIs in treatment of SSD with mixed results [32], fluoxetine, sertraline, and fluvoxamine have shown efficacy in the treatment of other paraphilias, especially in mild cases involving juveniles or those with comorbid depressive or OCD symptoms [33, 34]. However, controlled trials are still absent from the current literature [28].

Antiandrogen treatments, such as medroxyprogesterone acetate (MPA) or cyproterone acetate (CPA), have both progestogenic and antiandrogenic effects, which serve to decrease both dihydrotestosterone and testosterone. While CPA is available in most countries, MPA has been the agent of choice within the United States though it has largely been abandoned in Europe due to poor risk/benefit ratio, as discussed below [28]. Both medications are available in depot preparations.

MPA shows efficacy; reduction or complete disappearance of deviant sexual fantasies and behavior were observed after 1–2 months in the majority of cases [35–37]. With depot preparations, recidivism in MPA was 27 % (compared to 50 % before treatment) and was greater than with the use of CPA [38]. MPA is also associated with severe side effects including but not limited to pulmonary embolism, weight gain, diabetes mellitus, and Cushing syndrome [28].

CPA is associated with significant decrease in patient-reported sexual fantasies and activity, and in 80–90 % of cases within 1–3 months shows complete remission of deviant sexual behavior and remained efficacious as long as the treatment as continued [39–41]. Re-offense rate with CPA was found to be 6 % (lower than CPA as previously mentioned), as compared with 85 % before therapy [38]. The side effect profile for CPA is similar to MPA.

GnRH analogues, including triptorelin and leuprorelin work by causing a desensitization in GnRH receptors, which leads to a decrease in luteinizing hormone and a subsequent decrease of testosterone to castrate levels within 2–4 weeks [28]. This is after an initially stimulatory period which actually increases testosterone. In studies, CPA or flutamide were often used during the initial treatment with GnRH analogues to counter this stimulatory period.

Studies with triptorelin have shown the medication to be very successful; of 75 subjects across three studies, deviant sexual behavior was completely abolished in all but one patient despite the studied group containing patients who previously failed a trial with CPA [42–44]. Leuoprorelin showed similar efficacy to triptorelin across multiple studies [45–47] leading to a disappearance in deviant sexual behavior and fantasies in more than 90 % of cases after 1–3 months of therapy.

Side effects for these medications include bone mineral loss which requires biyearly monitoring and possible calcium, vitamin D, or bisphosphonate supplementation [48], hot flashes, asthenia, nausea, weight gain, decreased facial and body hair growth, decreased glucose tolerance, decreased testicular volume, depressive symptoms, and mild gynecomastia. However, when appropriately prescribed with careful follow-up and treatment of side effects, these medications are well tolerated and similar in risk to many other forms of frequently prescribed medications [49].

Cognitive behavioral therapy has been a mainstay treatment of sexual offenders and should focus on criminogenic factors rather than cognitive distortions or trying to have patients take full responsibility for their offense [50]. The practitioner should focus on important factors that lead to future criminal behavior including relationship difficulties, poor self-regulation, sexually deviant interests, and preoccupations, and a limited set of cognitive distortions excluding denial, minimizations, excuses, and justifications which all fail to predict reoffending [51, 52].

Conclusion

Sexual sadism disorder presents numerous challenges: defining it so that it has clinical utility while not being overly inclusive, identifying individuals with the disorder who pose the largest risk of offending and who most require treatment, and then maintaining them on that treatment despite significant side effects. The literature on the disorder is limited mainly to male forensic populations and often has required self-reporting, which is less than ideal with regard to a disorder that is heavily negatively connoted. However, criteria other than DSM-5 or ICD-10, such as the SSSS or SORAG, may offer better predictive value or diagnostic ability than using self-reports alone. As well, newer medications in the form of GnRH agonists provide promise of better outcomes with fewer and more easily managed side effects than older antiandrogen standbys. None the less, the disorder represents both a diagnostic and treatment challenge to practitioners.

References

1. Briken P, Bourget D, Dufour M. Sexual sadism in sexual offenders and sexually motivated homicide. Psychiatr Clin North Am. 2014;37(2):215–30. doi:10.1016/j.psc.2014.03.003.
2. Marshall WL, Hucker SJ, McAnulty RD, Burnette MM. Severe sexual sadism: its features and treatment. In: Sex and sexuality, Sexual deviation and sexual offenses, vol. 3. Westport: Praeger; 2006. p. 227–50.
3. World Health Organization. Tenth revision of the International Classification of Diseases, chapter V (F): mental and behavioural disorders. Diagnostic criteria for research. Geneva: World Health Organization; 1993.

4. American Psychiatric Association. Diagnostic and statistical manual of mental disorders. 5th ed. Arlington: American Psychiatric Publishing; 2013. p. 685–705.
5. American Psychiatric Association. Diagnostic and statistical manual of mental disorder. 3rd ed., rev. Washington, DC: American Psychiatric Association; 1987.
6. American Psychiatric Association. Diagnostic and statistical manual of mental disorder. 4th ed. Washington, DC: American Psychiatric Association; 1994.
7. American Psychiatric Association. Diagnostic and statistical manual of mental disorder. 4th ed., text rev. Washington, DC: American Psychiatric Association; 2000.
8. Abel GG. Paraphilias. In: Kaplan HI, Sadock BJ, editors. Comprehensive textbook of psychiatry, vol. 1. 5th ed. Baltimore: Williams & Williams; 1989. p. 1069–89.
9. Knight RA, Prentky RA. Classifying sexual offenders: the development and corroboration of taxonomic models. In: Marshall WL, Law DL, Barbaree HE, editors. Handbook of sexual assault: issues, theories and treatment of the offender. New York: Plenum; 1990. p. 23–52.
10. Knight RA, Prentky RA, Cerce DD. The development, reliability, and validity of an inventory for the multidimensional assessment of sex and aggression. Crim Justice Behav. 1994;21:72–94.
11. Marshall WL, Kennedy P. Sexual sadism in sexual offenders: an elusive diagnosis. Aggress Violent Behav. 2003;8:1–22.
12. Dietz PE, Hazelwood RR, Warren J. The sexually sadistic criminal and his offenses. Bull Am Acad Psychiatry Law. 1990;18:163–78.
13. Richards H, Jackson RL. Behavioral discriminators of sexual sadism and paraphilia nonconsent in a sample of civilly committed sexual offenders. Int J Offender Ther Comp Criminol. 2011;55(2):207–27.
14. Berner W, Berger P, Hill A. Sexual sadism. Int J Offender Ther Comp Criminol. 2003;47:383–95.
15. Eher R, Schilling F, Hansmann BT. Sexual sadism and violent reoffending in sexual offenders. Paper presented at ATSA conference. October 30–November 2, 2013, Chicago, IL, USA.
16. Bourget D, Bradford JM. Evidential basis for the assessment and treatment of sex offenders. Brief Treat Crisis Interv. 2008;8:130–46.
17. Healey J, Lussier P, Beauregard E. Sexual sadism in the context of rape and sexual homicide: an examination of crime scene indicators. Int J Offender Ther Comp Criminol. 2012;57:402–24.

18. Larue D, Schmidt AF, Imhoff R, et al. Validation of direct and indirect measure of preference for sexualized violence. Psychol Assess. 2014;26(4):1173–83.
19. Mokros A, Schilling F, Eher R, et al. The severe sexual sadism scale: cross validation and scale properties. Psychol Assess. 2012;24:764–9.
20. Marshall WL, Kennedy P, Yates P, et al. Diagnosing sexual sadism in sexual offenders: reliability across diagnosticians. Int J Offender Ther Comp Criminol. 2002;46:668–77.
21. Marshall WL, Hucker SJ. Issues in the diagnosis of sexual sadism. Sexual offender treatment I. 2006. http://www.sexual-offender-treatment.org/40.html#top. Accessed 11 Jan 2013.
22. Kingston DA, Seto MC, Firestone P, et al. Comparing indicators of sexual sadism as predictors of recidivism among adult male sexual offenders. J Consult Clin Psychol. 2010;78:574–84.
23. Quinsey VL, Harris GT, Rice ME, et al. Violent offenders: appraising and managing risk. 2nd ed. Washington, DC: American Psychological Association; 2006.
24. Hare RD. The hare psychopathy checklist-revised. Toronto: Multi-Health Systems; 1991.
25. Krueger RB. The DSM, diagnostic criteria for sexual sadism. Arch Sex Behav. 2010;39:325–45.
26. Eher R, Rettenberger M, Schilling F. Psychiatrische Diagnosen von Sexualstraftatern: Eine empirische Untersuchung von 807 inhaftierten Kindesmissbrauchsta tern und Vergewaltigern. [Psychiatric diagnoses of sexual offenders. An empirical study of 807 incarcerated child abuse offenders and rapists]. Z Sexualforsch. 2010;23:23–35.
27. Mokros A, Schilling F, Weiss K, et al. Sadism in sexual offenders: evidence for dimensionality. Psychol Assess. 2014;26:138–47.
28. Thibaut F. Pharmacological treatment of paraphilias. Isr J Psychiatry Relat Sci. 2012;49(4):297–305.
29. Garcia F, Thibaut F. Current concepts in the pharmacotherapy of paraphilias. Drugs. 2011;71:771–90.
30. Hanson RK, Morton-Bourgon KE. The characteristics of persistent sexual offenders: a meta-analysis of recidivism studies. J Consult Clin Psychol. 2005;73:1154–63.
31. Thibaut F, Torres de la Barra F, Gordon H, Bradford JMW, Cosyns P, the WFSBP Task Force on Sexual Disorders. The World Federation of Societies of Biological Psychiatry (WFSBP) guidelines for the biological treatment of paraphilias. World J Biol Psychiatry. 2010;11:604–55.

32. Casals-Ariet C, Cullen K. Exhibitionism treated with clomipramine. Am J Psychiatry. 1993;150:1273–4.
33. Kafka MP. Sertraline pharmacotherapy for paraphilias and paraphiliarelated disorders: an open trial. Ann Clin Psychiatry. 1994;6:189–95.
34. Bradford J, Fedoroff P. Pharmacological treatment of the juvenile sex offender. In: Barbaree H, Marshall W, editors. The juvenile sex offender. 2nd ed. New York: Guilford; 2006. p. 358–82. Chapter 16.
35. Wincze JP, Bansal S, Malamud M. Effects of medroxyprogesterone acetate on subjective arousal, arousal to erotic stimulation, and nocturnal penile tumescence in male sex offenders. Arch Sex Behav. 1986;15:293–305.
36. Hucker S, Langevin R, Bain J. A double-blind trial of sex drive reducing medication in pedophiles. Ann Sex Res. 1988;1:227–47.
37. Kiersch TA. Treatment of sex offenders with Depo Provera. Bull Am Acad Psychiatry Law. 1990;18:179–87.
38. Meyer JW, Cole CM. Physical and chemical castration of sex offenders: a review. J Off Rehab. 1997;25:1–18.
39. Cooper AJ. A placebo controlled trial of the antiandrogen cyproterone acetate in deviant hypersexuality. Compr Psychiatry. 1981;22:458–65.
40. Bradford JM, Pawlak A. Double-blind placebo crossover study of cyproterone acetate in the treatment of the paraphilias. Arch Sex Behav. 1993;22:383–402.
41. Cooper AJ, Cernovsky Z. The effects of cyproterone acetate on sleeping and waking penile erections in pedophiles: possible implications for treatment. Can J Psychiatry. 1992;37:33–9.
42. Thibaut F, Cordier B, Kuhn JM. Effect of a long-lasting gonodatrophin hormone-releasing hormone agonist in six cases of severe male paraphilia. Acta Psychiatr Scand. 1993;87:445–50.
43. Thibaut F, Cordier B, Kuhn J. Gonadotrophin hormone releasing hormone agonist in cases of severe paraphilia: a lifetime treatment? Psychoneuroendocrinology. 1996;21:411–9.
44. Rösler A, Witztum E. Treatment of men with paraphilia with a long-acting analogue of gonadotropin-releasing hormone. N Eng J Med. 1998;338:416–22.
45. Czerny JP, Briken P, Berner W. Antihormonal treatment of paraphilic patients in German forensic psychiatric clinics. Eur Psychiatry. 2002;17:104–6.

46. Briken P, Nika E, Berner W. Treatment of paraphilia with luteinizing hormone-releasing hormone agonists. J Sex Marital Ther. 2001;27:45–55.
47. Briken P. Pharmacotherapy of paraphilias with luteinizing hormonereleasing hormone agonists. Arch Gen Psychiatry. 2002;59:469–70.
48. Hoogeveen GH, Van Der Veer E. Side effects of pharmacotherapy on bone with long-acting gonadorelin agonist triptorelin for paraphilia. J Sex Med. 2008;5:626–30.
49. Berlin F. Sex offender treatment and legislation. J Am Acad Psychiatry Law. 2003;31:510–3.
50. Karl HR, Yates PM. Psychological treatment of sex offenders. Curr Psychiatry Rep. 2013;15(3):348. doi:10.1007/s11920-012-0348-x.
51. Marshall WL, Marshall LE, Kingston DA. Are the cognitive distortions of child molesters in need of treatment? J Sex Aggress. 2011;17:118–29.
52. Marshall WL, Marshall LE, Ware J. Cognitive distortions in sexual offenders: should they all be treatment targets? Sex Abuse ANZ. 2009;2:70–8.

Chapter 10
Pedophilic Disorder

Julia Machado Khoury, Marco Antônio Valente Roque, and Frederico Duarte Garcia

Introduction

From the legal and clinical view, a difference exists between pedophilic disorder and pedophilic acting. A subject with pedophilic disorders present fantasies, thoughts or sexual urges and exciting involving children, but do not necessarily perform pedophilic acts.

Although the pedophilic acting is currently considered a crime in many countries, the attraction of adults for children has been described as historical fact in many ancient societies. In Rome the existence of this behavior, particularly the hebephilia, was acceptable. In many other countries, hebephilia

J.M. Khoury, M.D. • M.A.V. Roque, M.D.
Department of Mental Health, Regional Center on Addictions (CRR-UFMG) and Post-graduation in Molecular Medicine of the Federal University of Minas Gerais (UFMG), Avenida Prof. Alfredo Balena, 190, Sala 240, Belo Horizonte, MG 30130, Brazil

F.D. Garcia, M.D., Ph.D. (✉)
Department of Mental Health, Regional Center on Addictions (CRR-UFMG) and Post-graduation in Molecular Medicine of the Federal University of Minas Gerais (UFMG), Avenida Prof. Alfredo Balena, 190, Sala 240, Belo Horizonte, MG 30130, Brazil

Inserm Unity 1073, Rouen University, Mont-Saint-Aignan, France
e-mail: frederico.garcia@gmail.com; fredgarcia@ufmg.br

R. Balon (ed.), *Practical Guide to Paraphilia and Paraphilic Disorders*, DOI 10.1007/978-3-319-42650-1_10

or even pedophilia was also tolerated. For this reason, in 1989, the United Nations approved the International Convention on the Rights of the Child that, in its article 19, expressly forces the states to adopt measures to protect children and adolescents from abuse, threat, or injury to their sexual integrity.

The 5th Edition of the Diagnostic and Statistical Manual of Mental Disorders (DSM 5) [1] classified pedophilia as a paraphilic disorder and the World Health Organization in 10th Edition of the International Classification of Diseases as a sexual preference disorder [2].

Pedophilia is a chronical condition that usually begins in youth or the beginning of adulthood and persists throughout life [3, 4]. This disorder is characterized by behaviors, fantasies and/or recurring sexual thoughts, intense and exciting involving children of up to 12 years old, over a period, equal or superior to 6 months [1]. The patient with a pedophilic disorder can be attracted to girls only, boys only, or children of both genders [1, 2].

The pedophilic disorder can only be diagnosed when a subject perceives that his attraction and sexual preference to children is producing psychosocial difficulties. If the subject conveys a lack of guilt, shame, or anxiety towards these urges, he has no functional limitation, and he has never practiced these urges, this person has pedophilic sexual orientation and not pedophilic disorder [1].

The prevalence of the pedophilic disorder is unknown, although some authors estimate a prevalence of 3–5 % with a higher prevalence predominance among males [1]. The evolution of the disorder tend to oscillate, with an increase of the urges in adolescence, and young adulthood and a decrease with age [1], this is probably correlated with testosterone levels.

Diagnostic Criteria

Clinical assessment of a patient with a pedophilic disorder comprise the sexual anamnesis and the exam of the mental state [5]. Sexual anamnesis is important because it provides detailed information regarding sexual activities, preferences and, pornography use. The intense use of child pornography is considered a major risk factor for engaging in sexual aggression, as the subject tends to prefer pornographic types in correspondence to their sexual interests [1, 6]. The diagnostic criteria for the pedophilic disorder according to the DSM 5 are [1] (Reprinted with permission from the diagnostic and Statistical Manual of Mental Disorders, Fifth Edition, (Copyright 2013). American Psychiatric Association):

(a) *Over a period of at least 6 months, recurrent, intense sexually arousing fantasies, sexual urges, or behaviors involving sexual activity with a prepubescent child or children (generally 13 years or younger).*
(b) *The individual has acted on these sexual urges, or the sexual urges or fantasies cause marked distress or interpersonal difficulty.*
(c) *The individual is at least, 16 years and at least 5 years older than the child or children in Criterion.*

Note: Do not include an individual in late adolescence involved in an ongoing sexual relationship with 12- or 13-year-old.
Specify whether:
Exclusive type (attracted only to children)
Nonexclusive type
Specify if:
Sexually attracted to males
Sexually attracted to females
Sexually attracted to both
Specify if:
Limited to incest.

The pedophilic disorder is the only paraphilic disorder (except "Other specified paraphilic disorder" and "Not specified paraphilic disorder") that does not possess the specifiers "in a protected environment" and "in complete remission." The specifier "in a protected environment" (available to the diagnosis criteria of the Voyeuristic, Exhibitionist, Frotteurism, Sexual Masochism, Sexual Sadism, Fetish and Transvestic disorders) applies to institutionalized individuals or residents of other locations where the opportunity of involvement in paraphilic behaviors could be restricted. The specifier "in complete remission" indicates that the individual has not put into practice the urges with a person who has not consented, and there was no distress or impairment in social, occupational, or other areas of the individual's life for at least 5 years while in an unprotected environment. The lack of these two specifiers for the paraphilic disorder may reflect the stigma the controversies that surround political decisions regarding paraphilic disorders [7]. The specifier that makes reference to the protected environment could be useful on the approach of patients with a paraphilic disorder as it may gauge the propensity of an individual to impulsively act when he has no opportunity to act on this urge [7]. Regarding the absence of the "in complete remission" specifier, may be misinterpreted as if the subject suffering from pedophilic disorder would never reach remission. This fact is currently not supported by the literature and can cause serious political and legal consequences, increasing, even more, the stigma over mental health disorders [7].

Psychophysiological measures of the sexual interest can be useful when there is a suspicion of pedophilic disorder, but the patient denies the symptoms. Among the examinations utilized, we can mention the penile plethysmograph, which measures the sexual attraction for children through the measuring of penis erection, and the visualization time, which uses pictures of naked or semi-naked children as a visual stimulus [1].

The use of naked or minimally dressed children images in the "penile plethysmography" and in "display time" as psychophysiological measures of the sexual interest for the diagnosis of pedophilic disorder is controversial and legally risky. In many countries, child pornography is illegal and therefore considered a punishable crime, including incarceration. Therefore, professionals of mental health and researchers should be aware that the possession of such visual stimulus, even for diagnostic purposes, may violate the laws exposing these professionals to criminal prosecution.

Differential diagnoses for the paraphilic disorder includes the cluster B personality disorders, especially the antisocial personality disorder, which may favor the pedophilic sexual behavior because of impulsive traits or based on the relative availability. These individuals often show other signs of personality disorders, such as recurrent disregard for the laws, a dysfunctional pattern of interpersonal relationships, and strict general operating standards.

Another differential diagnosis comprises substance use disorders, mainly the use of alcohol and other psychoactive substances, which increase the likelihood of sexual attraction to children by disinhibited effects of intoxication. Therefore, it is important to assess actively the use of these substances and the pattern of use. The pedophilic disorder can coexist as long as the sexual attraction to children and pedophile behavior is not restricted to periods of intoxication.

The pedophile disorder may also be confused with obsessive compulsive disorder (OCD). Some individuals with OCD diagnosis complain of egodystonic thoughts and concerns about sexual attraction to children or images of naked children. Unlike OCD, generally, sexual attraction to children in pedophilic disorder is egosyntonic. In addition, the OCD anamnesis may reveal other egodystonic intrusive sexual ideas and absence of sexual thoughts about children during sexual excitation states, such as orgasm and masturbation.

Summary of Evidence

The etiology of the paraphilic disorder remains poorly understood, but the current literature points towards the involvement of neurological, hormonal, and psychodynamic alterations.

The neurological modification already described are unspecific and comprise a considerable decrease of the volume of the gray matter of the right amygdala, the hypothalamus, the septal area, the innominate substance, and the nucleus of the stria terminalis. These alterations may reflect environmental aggression at critical periods of psychosexual development [8]. Moreover, one study reported changes in the cortico-striatal-thalamic-cortical circuit of these subjects and a decrease of the ventral striatum nucleus, the orbitofrontal cortex, and cerebellum. These brain modifications have been related to impulsive and aggressive personality traces [9].

The studies assessing EEG alterations report an abnormal increase of the alpha rhythm and a decrease in the frontal areas in patients with pedophilia exposed to children images [10].

Patients with a pedophilic disorder present may show a partial disconnection of the net that connects the occiput posterior frontal lobe and the arcuate fasciculus with the cortical areas activated by the visual sexual stimulus, as shown in functional magnetic resonance studies [8, 11].

Other studies describe an increase in testosterone levels and the luteinizing hormone in patients with the pedophilic disorder, mostly in those subjects with an aggressive personality trace [12, 13], which may indicate a hypothalamic-pituitary-gonadal axis dysfunction.

The antisocial personality disorder can be considered a risk factor for the pedophilic disorder in men [1]. The sexual and/or emotional abuse in the childhood were also associated with pedophilia in the adulthood [1, 5], as well as having belonged to large families and being the son of older parents [13]. There are some evidence that the disturbance of the neurodevelopment in the intrauterine life increases the possibility of pedophile orientation development [1].

Many studies have shown consistently high rates of psychiatric comorbidity in patients with paraphilias. The most usual ones are the disorder by use of substances, especially alcohol, unipolar depressive disorder, bipolar disorder, anxiety disorders, antisocial personality disorder, mood disorder, and other paraphilic disorders [1, 13].

Clinical Case

Mr. W. is a 27-year-old man, referred by his general practitioner to the addiction center for the assessment of a possible sexual addiction. The patient described that he presented several

(7–8) episodes of masturbation in a day since he was 14 years old. During his interview, he stated "I was abused when I was little. I know how it can make someone suffer. I am now really distressed because I am afraid of doing the same with someone else and hurt him as I was hurt." He seeks help after quitting a stable heterosexual relationship because the women had a 10-year-old child. He reported that since the age of 16, he presented sexual fantasies with male children and in the last 6 months he was concerned about not being able to resist his urges and to acting out. His fantasies and urges produced intense shame, anxiety, and suffering. He denied previous sexual experiences with children and avoided the use of child pornography for personal and religious reasons. In past history, he described a previous depressive episode treated with fluoxetine 20 mg M.I.D., which was well tolerated. A maternal uncle suicided in an unclear situation, and his mother had a diabetes mellitus. Physical exam and laboratory assessment were normal. The patient accepted treatment with fluoxetine 20 mg, which was titrated up to 80 mg in 4 weeks. After 3 months of treatment, the patient referred a decrease in his sexual urges and pedophilic fantasies although, still feared to act out. Cognitive behavior therapy was hence initiated to aid him develop alternative thoughts and deal with self-esteem. After 12 months of treatment, fluoxetine was decreased to 40 mg and the patient was stable.

Recommendations

The therapeutic approaches for paraphilic disorders, including the pedophilic disorder, are controversial and are still based on the decrease of testosterone levels, and psychotherapeutic support [14, 15]. Due to the lack of strong evidence proving the efficacy or the superiority of any treatment, clinicians must consider these limitations when considering any treatment options here described. Some drugs recommended in the present recommendations are not available in all countries and approved doses may vary.

Clinical approaches should consider symptoms and treatment effectiveness [15].

Although surgical castration could be used to reduce testosterone and in consequence sexual urges, it is rarely practiced on these days due to legal and ethic aspects.

The individual and/or group psychotherapy, mostly through relapse prevention, behavioral, and cognitive approaches, is the treatment method more commonly used on paraphilic disorders [16].

However, evidence and medical consensus suggest that the best therapeutic strategies are those that combine psychotherapeutic and pharmacological treatment [17].

The pharmacotherapies are based on two main medications type: (1) antiandrogenic drugs, to reduce testosterone production or to antagonize its action; and (2) psychotropic drugs, such as the antidepressants [16].

Antiandrogenic Drugs

Testosterone is a sexual hormone crucial for the development of the male secondary sexual characteristics and has an important regulatory function on sexuality, cognition, emotion, personality, and aggressive behavior [16]. Testosterone also activates the sexual desire and erection [16].

Drugs that antagonize or decrease testosterone secretion preclude its action and results in a reduction in sexual desire or pedophilic behavior.

Currently, it is suggested that these drugs must be utilized for long term since the therapeutic effects last for only a few months after the use interruption.

The main antiandrogenic medications for the treatment of pedophilic disorder treatment are:

1. Cyproterone acetate
2. Medroxyprogesterone acetate
3. Analogs of long-acting gonadotropin release (GnRGH) [16]

The primary secondary effects are gynecomastia, weakness, weight gain, thromboembolism, depression, liver damage, a decrease of pilosity, a decrease in bone mineral density, nightmares, headaches, dyspepsia, diabetes mellitus, and a decrease of testicular volume [16].

Psychotropic Drugs

High doses of selective serotonin reuptake inhibitors (SSRI) may decrease sexual fantasies and urges, impulsivity and the capacity of erection, regardless of the presence of comorbidity with depressive and anxiety disorders. However, there is no evidence on the effectiveness of these drugs in the treatment of patients with paraphilic disorders treatment [16–18].

Lithium carbonate, tricyclic antidepressants (clomipramine and desipramine), antipsychotics (benperidol, thioridazine, haloperidol), and anticonvulsants (carbamazepine) have also been tested for the treatment of patients with paraphilic disorders, although no evidence proves the efficacy of these drugs in the disorder [18].

Chemical Castration

The treatment of patients with the paraphilic disorder has always been controversial and the subject of clinical and ethical dilemmas. The biggest ethical dilemma is the dispute between the need for public safety/punishment and effectiveness/treatment indication [19–21]. Patients with the pedophilic disorder are often targets of coercion (by justice, by family, and others) to submit themselves to treatment by castration, especially when other treatments have not proven effective.

Chemical castration has emerged as a possible therapy for pedophilic disorder, considering that it is the use of medications to control sexual impulses and inhibit the libido of individuals with this condition. Therefore, it acts to inhibit libido and hence the possibility of sexual intercourse. From an ethical point of view, patients can undergo chemical castration only if all the following criteria are met [22]:

- The disorder was diagnosed by a psychiatrist after careful psychiatric examination
- The castration should specifically target the clinical signs, symptoms, and behaviors and treatment should be adapted to the health conditions of the individual
- The individual's condition represents a significant risk of serious injury to his health or physical/moral integrity of others
- Any other form of treatment less intrusive is available or was effective
- The psychiatrist that assists the individual agrees to inform him about the risks and benefits and receive his consent, as well as being responsible for the indication of treatment and its follow-up
- The castration is part of a written treatment plan that should be reviewed at appropriate intervals and, if necessary, restructured

Chemical castration has been applied as a penalty for those judged pedophiles in various countries like Canada, Wales, and several US states [23]. It is a procedure that has many clinical and ethical limitations, and significant side effects. The hormonal castration is nothing more than a temporal chemical procedure, being its utilization variable. Although it is a reversible procedure, its side effects continue to have importance in the debate about its adoption. Exemplifying possible side effects resulting from medical castration, Ponteli and Sanches Jr. [24] highlight: cardiovascular disease, osteoporosis, depression, headaches, stroke, and others. Such adverse effects affect the individual both in physical/biological and the psychological/psychiatric sphere, positioning the medical castration as a "risky" procedure. There is also a known risk of relapse in subjects that, after castration, inject testosterone in themselves with the purpose of reducing side effects.

The surgical castration, on the other hand, is performed only in the few countries, such as Czech Republic, Switzerland, Germany, and some Asiatic countries [25]. In the Netherlands castration was the method of choice for all types of aggressive offenders, at least after World War II until the late 1960s. At the beginning of 1979, however, the Dutch government declared castration illegal for the treatment of institutionalized patients [26]. Currently, in countries where it is permitted, surgical castration is performed as a last resort and generally when the individual committed serious sexual crime [27]. It is contraindicated for schizophrenics sex offenders or patients with severe psychopathy [27]. The main side effects include weight gain, gynecomastia, reduced body hair, sweating, hot flashes, osteopenia and osteoporosis, body and headache pain, dizziness, breathing difficulties, depression, social isolation, passivity, decreased psychomotor energy [28]. The risk of committing a subsequent sexual crime is reduced for sex offenders after they are castrated and released. However, intervals between castration and recidivism range from 6 weeks to 20 years after release [28]. As in chemical castration, surgical castration may be reversed by self-administration of testosterone by the treated individuals.

Those who advocate against this procedure state that it clearly violates human rights and from an ethical point of view, the castration should be avoided as punishment. Although, some patients and clinicians argue that it could be used as a form of treatment for individuals suffering from a pedophilic disorder and/or pose a risk to others and who have not responded to other forms of treatment less invasive.

Conclusion

Pedophilia, when it causes alterations in the functionality or significant suffering, is considered a paraphilic disorder. This disorder is experienced by the patients at the beginning of their sexual lives and presents a chronic evolution. This condition is more frequent in men, and it is characterized by behaviors, recurrent, intense, and exciting sexual thoughts and/or fantasies involving children up to 12 years old, for a period equal or greater than 6 months. Furthermore, the individual must be, at least, 16 years old and be at least 5 years older than the child.

The etiology of this disorder remains poorly clarified, but the current literature suggests the involvement of possible neurological, hormonal, and psychodynamic alterations. The treatment includes surgical, psychotropic, and pharmacological techniques. The medications most utilized are the antiandrogenic drugs and the psychotropic drugs. Future controlled studies are warranted to improve evidence regarding efficacy and duration of the pharmacologic treatment.

Acknowledgements
This paper was supported by FAPEMIG (Fundação de Pesquisa do Estado de Minas Gerais, Brazil) under grant APQ-01714-13 and the National Conceal for Scientific and Technological Development, CNPq (Conselho Nacional de Desenvolvimento Tecnológico, Brazil) under grant 486221/2013-0.

References

1. American Psychiatric Association. The diagnostic and statistical manual of mental disorders. 5th ed. Arlington: American Psychiatric Association; 2013.
2. World Health Organization. International statistical classification of diseases and health related problems (The) ICD-10. Diss. Geneva: World Health Organization; 2004.
3. Quinsey VL. The etiology of anomalous sexual preferences in men. Ann N Y Acad Sci. 2003;989:105–17; 144–53.
4. Studer LH, Aylwin AS. Pedophilia: the problem with diagnosis and limitations of CBT in treatment. Med Hypotheses. 2006;67(4):774–81.
5. Hughes JR. Review of medical reports on pedophilia. Clin Pediatr (Phila). 2007;46(8):667–82.
6. Seto MC, Cantor JM, Blanchard R. Child pornography offenses are a valid diagnostic indicator of pedophilia. J Abnorm Psychol. 2006;115(3):610–5.
7. Balon R. Politics of diagnostic criteria: specifiers of pedophilic disorder in DSM-5. Arch Sex Behav. 2014;43(7):1235–6.
8. Walter M, Witzel J, Wiebking C, et al. Pedophilia is linked to reduced activation in hypothalamus and lateral prefrontal cor-

tex during visual erotic stimulation. Biol Psychiatry. 2007;62(6):698–701.
9. Schiltz K, Witzel J, Northoff G, et al. Brain pathology in pedophilic offenders: evidence of volume reduction in the right amygdala and related diencephalic structures. Arch Gen Psychiatry. 2007;64(6):737–46.
10. Schiffer B, Peschel T, Paul T, et al. Structural brain abnormalities in the frontostriatal system and cerebellum in pedophilia. J Psychiatr Res. 2007;41(9):753–62.
11. Schiffer B, Krueger T, Paul T, et al. Brain response to visual sexual stimuli in homosexual pedophiles. J Psychiatry Neurosci. 2008;33(1):23–33.
12. Cantor JM, Kabani N, Christensen BK, et al. Cerebral white matter deficiencies in pedophilic men. J Psychiatr Res. 2008;42(3):167–83.
13. Rösler A, Witztum E. Pharmacotherapy of paraphilias in the next millennium. Behav Sci Law. 2000;18(1):43–56.
14. Saleh FM, Guidry LL. Psychosocial and biological treatment considerations for the paraphilic and nonparaphilic sex offender. J Am Acad Psychiatry Law. 2003;31(4):486–93.
15. Assumpção AA, Garcia FD, Garcia HD, Bradford JM, Thibaut F. Pharmacologic treatment of paraphilias. Psychiatr Clin North Am. 2014;37(2):173–81.
16. Garcia FD, Delavenne HG, Assupção AA, Thibaut F. Pharmacologic treatment of sex offenders with paraphilic disorder. Curr Psychiatry Rep. 2013;15(5):351.
17. Garcia FD, Thibaut F. Current Concepts in the parmacoterapy of paraphilias. Drugs. 2011;71(6):771–90.
18. Thibaut F, De La Barra F, Grodon H, Cosyns P, Bradford JM. WFSBP task force on sexual disorders. World J Biol Psychiatry. 2010;11(4):604–55.
19. Bowden P. Treatment: use, abuse and consent. Crim Behav Ment Health. 1991;1:130–41.
20. Ward T, Gannon TA, Brigden A. Human rights and the treatment of sex offenders. Sex Abuse. 2007;19:195–216.
21. Elger BS. REsearch involving prisioners: consensus and controversies in international and European regulation. Bioethics. 2008;22(4):224–38.
22. Belgian Advisory Committee on Bioethics 2006 [www.health.fgov.be/bioeth]; Council of Europe 2004.

23. Scott CL, Holmberg T. Castration of sex offenders: prisoners' rights versus public safety. J Am Acad Psychiatry Law. 2003;31(4):502–9. Accessed 6 Oct 2011.
24. Ponteli NN, Sanches Jr CA. Notes for a sociological analysis of the chemical castration. Rev Levs/Unesp. 2010;(5). http://www2.marilia.unesp.br/revistas/index.php/levs/article/viewFile/1111/999. Accessed 26 ago 2011.
25. Plenge H. Die Behandlung erheblich rtickf~illiger Sexualdelinquenten, vornehmlich der Homosexuellen, unter Beriicksichtigung der Kastration. Monatsschr Kriminol Strafreehtsreform. 1961;44:15–41.
26. Heim N. Sexual behavior of castrated sex offenders. Arch Sex Behav. 1981;10(1):11–9.
27. Langeltiddeke A. Castration of sexual criminals. Berlin: de Gruyter; 1963.
28. Heim N, Hursch CJ. Castration for sex offenders: treatment or punishment? A review and critique of recent European literature. Arch Sex Behav. 1979;8(3):281–304.

Chapter 11
Fetishistic Disorder

Scott F. Martin

Introduction

Fetishistic disorder is a DSM-5 recognized paraphilic disorder that is less likely to involve illegal behavior or victimization, but is essential in characterizing the versatility of the human sexual imagination. This disorder is demarcated by a distressing and persisting pattern of sexual arousal involving the use of nonliving objects or atypical, nongenital body parts. In the field of cultural anthropology, the term fetish refers to idols and talismans that have symbolic religious meaning. In medical usage the term delineates an object, commonly an item of clothing, which is used by an individual to attain sexual arousal and orgasm. Sexual fetishists frequently need to be touching, smelling, or looking at their unique object, or engaging in fantasy about it in order to function sexually alone or with a partner. Like the religious fetish, the sexual fetish can have significant meaning, but it is a meaning held only by the individual and is not shared by the larger community.

S.F. Martin, M.D. (✉)
Department of Psychiatry, Case Western Reserve University School of Medicine, Center for Marital and Sexual Health,
23425 Commerce Park Rd., Suite 104, Beachwood, OH 44122, USA
e-mail: smartinmd@gmail.com

R. Balon (ed.), *Practical Guide to Paraphilia and Paraphilic Disorders*, DOI 10.1007/978-3-319-42650-1_11

Fetishism has been recognized as a sexual variation for over 100 years, and has very often been considered a disorder in all of its presenting forms. Recent and ongoing social developments through the exposure of the internet have confirmed the high incidence of fetishistic behavior. We see eccentric behaviors that are met with acceptance by online communities of like minded individuals, and ready availability of means for adaptation and integration into the mental and sexual lives of individuals so affected. Clinical distress of affected individuals, when present and persisting, can now be highlighted as an essential diagnostic feature of fetishistic disorder, and can be considered as a potential target for treatment.

Even when accompanied by high levels of distress, fetishistic disorder remains a rare patient presenting complaint. Fetishists may not understand it to be an appropriate target of medical intervention, or they may be embarrassed to discuss their requirement for arousal, especially if a psychiatrist or other physician has not created a comfortable environment for the discussion of sexual matters.

Research into fetishistic disorder also remains rare. The focus of research has been on the specific diagnostic criteria needed to define this condition as a disorder, and on making rudimentary estimations of prevalence in the general population. The evidence for understanding and treating fetishistic disorder is largely based on clinical experience and on case studies, but not on controlled trials.

Diagnostic Criteria

The descriptive terminology of atypical sexual behavior has included Fetishism since the early twentieth century, and is included in the writings of Freud and of Binet, Krafft-Ebing, and Ellis before him [1]. This early usage of the term fetishism did not refer distinctly to pathological behavior but to a form of eroticization that lay on a continuum from pathological to normal. Early use of the term also included body parts and body products as the object of eroticization. Current DSM terminology has evolved and now DSM-5 has reincorporated the use of nongenital body parts, previously referred to as Partialism.

DSM-5 has also clarified the terminology, allowing again for the term fetishism to refer to the non pathological presence of particular erotic urges or behaviors, but specifying that fetishistic disorder be used for the uniquely pathological entity where a clinical level of distress is experienced by the patient.

The current DSM-5 criteria are as follows (Reprinted with permission from the Diagnostic and Statistical Manual of Mental Disorders, Fifth Edition, (Copyright 2013). American Psychiatric Association):

- *Over a period of at least 6 months, recurrent and intense sexual arousal from either the use of nonliving objects or a highly specific focus on nongenital body part(s), as manifested by fantasies, urges, or behaviors.*
- *The fantasies, sexual urges, or behaviors cause clinically significant distress or impairment in social, occupational, or other important areas of functioning.*
- *The fetish objects are not limited to articles of clothing used in cross-dressing (as in transvestic disorder) or devices designed for the purpose of tactile genital stimulation (e.g., vibrator) [2].*

The focus on body products remains absent from the criteria. A new challenge with the inclusion of nongenital body parts is how to delineate the pathological (from toes and feet to ankles to more traditionally eroticized areas such as legs, hips, buttocks, breasts, and hair). Criterion B, clinical distress, remains a crucial consideration in separating pathology from variations in normal expression.

Diagnostic accuracy requires that fetishistic disorder not be mistaken for an undefined paraphilic disorder, despite common usage of the term fetishism in referring to any unusual (and not otherwise categorized) sexual behavior. The eroticization of animals or of body products does not constitute fetishistic behavior, nor would an excessive focus on genital parts such as breasts, even if the behavior or fantasy interfered with partnered sexual functioning. There is also a differentiation to be made between an erotic focus on an object or use of that object, and an eroticization of more complex behaviors, such as solitary or partnered role-play, that utilizes certain objects. This is a distinction between the object itself and the meaning of the object to the individual, or the way in which it is incorporated into the erotic imagination, and may offer guidance in considering treatments.

Clinical Case Example

A man who is singularly sexually aroused by cowboy fantasies is filled with sexual energy upon smelling or even imagining the smell of the leather holster or boots that he utilizes in masturbatory behaviors. The handling and smelling of these objects is sufficient for him to achieve full sexual arousal. However, the fantasy gets played out much further and includes hours of reading the stories of outlaws, dressing and acting the role of outlaws, and finally imagining their hangings or engaging in an autoerotic asphyxiation routine that can culminate in ejaculation free from tactile stimulation. The role play and masturbation are always solitary and require the use of these or other similar objects, but the elements of ruthless behavior and of hanging, in addition to the wearing of costumes and acting out of fantasy roles, all add to the erotic charge. This man wishes that he could rid himself of this elaborate sexual interest, and has many times destroyed his props and vowed never to repeat the behavior. He has tremendous guilt and fear of being discovered, possibly in an asphyxiated state despite the precautions that he takes.

Due to this significant level of distress in combination with the required use of these specific objects, fetishistic disorder is appropriately diagnosed, but comorbid would be multiple undefined paraphilias that include the outlaw fantasy and role playing, the hanging fantasy and asphyxiation behavior, and the accompanying sadistic and masochistic elements. This patient has benefitted from a supportive psychotherapy and has increasing periods of self-described "sobriety," but the urges and behaviors return, in a form similar to when they developed in his adolescence decades prior.

A recent examination of the Adult Baby Diaper League has also confirmed the distinction between the fetishist's sexual excitement elicited solely from wearing a diaper, in private or concealed, and more elaborate erotic role-play [3].

This latter behavior, endorsed by some but not all of Adult Baby Diaper League respondents, requires diapers to be worn by the fetishist but also holds essential the parenting behaviors, for some caring and containing and for others shaming and sadomasochistic. Of note, a minority of respondents (13 % of males, 9 % of females) reported ever having a period of more than 6 months when their fetishistic interests caused them problems or distress.

One must proceed carefully when making a diagnosis based upon behaviors that are considered "unusual." Cultural norms play a role in our understanding of health and illness, and have unavoidable impact on our definitions of disease. In addition, cultural norms may contribute to a patient's distress if their behavior is not socially acceptable and considered "deviant" or "perverted." In the area of sexual medicine, homosexuality and masturbation are both examples of behaviors that were historically considered disorders based upon their status as socially unacceptable. In fetishistic disorder, as the DSM criteria indicate, the distinction must be made between those with varying degrees of sexual interest in a fetish object and those who are significantly distressed or facing psychosocial impairment due to a disorder.

Summary of Evidence

Evidence for the characteristics of fetishistic disorder comes only from several sources, most of which cannot be generalized to the entire population.

The forensic population of psychiatric patients is commonly evaluated for sexual crimes involving the paraphilias. The conditions primarily seen are Pedophilic, Exhibitionistic and Voyeuristic, and Frotteuristic disorders, and while comorbid cases of fetishistic disorder exist, they are relatively uncommon amongst sexual offenders and rarely the focus of clinical intervention [4].

Evaluation and treatment of gender dysphoria frequently reveals cases of transvestic disorder, which differs from fetishistic disorder as defined above but which also includes overlap or comorbidity of conditions. Blanchard investigated

247 males who reported transvestism (sexual arousal from dressing in women's clothing) and found that 60.3 % of them also met the independent criteria for fetishistic disorder [5].

Evaluations of subsets of populations, for example, Weinberg et al. who surveyed a group of self-described homosexual and bisexual foot fetishists called the "Foot Fraternity" [6]. This study included 262 individuals and reported primary and overlapping objects of sexual arousal to be clean feet (endorsed by 60 %), boots (52 %), and shoes (49 %). Socks were also found to be sexually arousing "a lot" of the time, notably with smelly socks being more often arousing than clean socks. This reflects their conclusion, based also upon answers to open-ended questions, that the fetish object induces a multi-sensory experience, including smell as well as taste, touch, and sight. A significant percent also emphasized the symbolism of the object as the primary source of arousal, in this case the symbolism of varying type and degrees of masculinity (boots vs. sneakers vs. wing-tips). Of particular diagnostic note in Weinberg's survey, 22.5 % of the individuals reported distress associated with their fetishistic interest, including loneliness, shame, and problems with intimate relationships. The conclusion here was that fetishism (as opposed to DSM-5 diagnosed fetishistic disorder) does not necessarily cause relationship or other psychosocial distress. Sixty percent of those surveyed were able to incorporate their interest in feet and/or footwear into their sexual lives with partners, with the remaining 17.5 % either satisfied to keep their interest secret from their partners or to confine their sexual lives to masturbation.

The largest assessment of atypical sexual interests self-defined as fetishistic is from Scorolli et al., who gathered data from English-language Yahoo internet discussion groups [7]. They reviewed message boards from 381 groups that included 150,000 total members, though recognizing that these anonymous individuals may belong to multiple groups. Their observation was of the sexual preferences expressed by these discussion participants. The participants were not assessed clinically and there was no means to assess whether they were distressed by their sexual interest (fetishistic disorder), but the results contribute to the evolving taxonomy. Scorolli et al. found the predominant sexual preferences to be for non-genital body parts and features (33 %) and objects associated with the body (30 %). Body parts were predominantly feet or toes (47 %) followed body fluids such as blood or urine (9 %), body features such as obesity or height, and hair, muscles, and body modifications such as tattoos and piercings. Objects associated with the body were those worn on the legs and buttocks such as stockings and skirts (33 %), footwear (32 %), whole-costumes, and less commonly stethoscopes, wristwatches, and diapers. Secondary preferences were expressed for the category "other people's behavior," such as smoking, and then "own behavior," "social behavior," and objects unrelated to the body (5 %). Internet studies have a presumed major sampling bias, but so do samples of psychiatric patients or arrested sexual offenders. It is unclear how these data reflect what exist in general populations and in various countries. The Internet is a new and evolving reflection of the variations in sexual behaviors, perhaps even impacting the development and flexibility of the sexual imagination.

Published clinical case studies, mostly in the psychoanalytic tradition, as well as the clinical experience of the author at the Center for Sexual and Marital Health, provide for additional observations that can be made regarding characteristics of fetishistic disorder. The following is a synthesis of those observations:

Fetishism presents almost exclusively in males. Theories as to why this is the case involve characteristic differences in power dynamics and expressions of control, gender prescribed outlets for initiating courtship and expressing attractiveness, and developmental variations in the flexibility and windows of fixity in establishment of erotic targets. Cases of fetishism in females have been reported [8], and a review of fetish oriented internet message boards reveals females in addition to males who are relieved to find that they are not alone in their variant sexual interests.

Fetishistic arousal patterns seem to be overrepresented in samples of men with significant developmental disabilities such as autism, intellectual deficiencies, and severe cerebral palsy. One must consider the effects of limited peer socialization as well as unknown direct biogenic causes in these situations. Temporal lobe dysfunction has been documented as a treatable cause in three cases of fetishistic disorder [9].

Fetishistic disorder is not diagnosed in children and rarely if ever in adolescents, though patients report that their unusual sexual interests were present from a young age. Abel et al. present cases where the object of sexual interest is unique enough for the patient, presenting in later years, to be able to trace back an initial presexual preoccupation or excitement in which the object (rings, cigarettes, feet) figured prominently [10]. It is usual for patients to recall an initial sexual preoccupation with the fetish object developing in adolescence during masturbation, either in the accompanying fantasies or the material objects held, caressed, or worn during penile stimulation.

In patients who present for treatment and who meet DSM criteria for a diagnosis of fetishistic disorder, the distress experienced is often in the realm of relationships. Unlike patients with strictly sadomasochistic paraphilic disorders, it is often more difficult for patients with fetishistic disorder to establish and maintain a place in their sexual relationship for their unique preoccupation. Ultimately, the fetish is not a shared object or interest, and what may begin for the partner as a curious or exciting oddity that they are willing to accommodate will very often be less welcome and precipitate conflict when the fetishist's sexual interest in the partner does not grow along with the relationship, but the excitement remains exclusively focused on the shoe or undergarments.

The interpersonal conflicts that develop in patients with fetishistic disorder commonly go beyond the functional difficulties described above and often reflect deeper disruptions of both identity and the ability to relate to others with a mature emotional intimacy [12]. Themes of control, power, and dehumanization often play important roles in the relationships of those with paraphilic disorders. Aggression towards a partner is rarely overt in fetishistic disorder, but the partner often feels hurt and may feel unloved or ashamed to find that their lover has sexual interest only in their toes or feet, and not in the partner as a whole emotional and sexual person. Theories (discussed below) do not agree on whether fetishistic disorder is a result or a cause of this further pathology.

Recommendations

Treatment of fetishistic disorder is without a strong evidence base, due in part to inadequate sample sizes. Psychotherapy is the primary accepted treatment modality, but can be time intensive and does not necessarily change the poor prognosis. Psychoanalysis has been used with reports of success, and psychodynamic psychotherapy is likewise thought to be beneficial, if not in altering the fetishistic preoccupation then in helping patients in the realm of relationship difficulties and in self-esteem and coherent identity development. Cognitive behavioral therapy and learning and conditioning theory may be employed in treatment but again have not been consistently proven effective. It is important to find a good fit between the presenting condition and a theory-driven treatment modality that is comfortable to both the clinician and patient.

Numerous theories have been advanced over the decades regarding the mechanisms that come into play in the development and persistence of fetishism and fetishistic disorder. The development of sexual identity in childhood, including the development of sexual intention that is disordered in fetishistic disorder, is not well understood. The psychoanalytic tradition has been the primary source of current theories, but more recently conditioning and social learning theory has also contributed.

Psychoanalytic thought tends to agree that the fetish object is utilized as an unconscious defense against anxiety. Freud found the source of this anxiety to be the confusion experienced during childhood at the realization of physical differences between the sexes, and the child's realization that the child does not have his mother to himself [8]. Termed castration anxiety, these feelings include but are not limited to the child's (and later adult's) ability to relate closely with others in the face of this potential (literal as well as figurative) loss. The over-investment in a fetish, according to the theory, is a compromise that allows an individual to function with a relatively coherent sense of identity, but with the limitations that the disorder entails.

Contemporary analytic theory agrees in large part with Freud's basic premise, but includes a wider variety of childhood emotional developments, and the accompanying anxieties provoked as painful feelings surface and are faced. Normal development requires learning to manage aggressive feelings, struggles with lack of control, separation from one's parents and the potential for loss of a parent's love. It is theorized that children who have less resilience, due to experiences with overwhelming abuse or neglect or to other disturbances to parental attachment, will struggle more in managing the normal sources of anxiety and will be more likely to develop a fetishistic disorder as compensation [12]. For example, the early struggles to manage separation from one's parents are commonly managed with the development of a transitional object, a blanket or toy, to which a child has a strong but temporary attachment. Fetishistic disorder can be understood in these terms as a more permanent attachment that less advantageously manages this developmental anxiety.

Abel utilizes conditioning theory to propose an alternative schema for understanding the fixation on a fetish object [10]. He suggests that early association of strong emotion with any given object can, if that object maintains a significance and becomes associated with the development of sexual arousal and masturbation, be reinforced with extensive repetition to the point that arousal cannot occur apart from that object, resulting in fetishistic disorder.

Blanchard also characterizes fetishistic disorder as a developmental disorder [13]. He proposes that it is a disorder of an individual's innate and differential sensitivity to various stimuli that, when combined with that individual's experience, may erroneously locate an erotic target that is oriented toward a "non-essential" feature of an ideally desired object (clothes rather than the person in the clothes).

The diagnostic criteria for fetishistic disorder provide little guidance for treatment and do not represent the variation that will be evident with clinical presentation. Clarifying the reason for presentation and characterizing the nature of the disorder will help clarify the target of treatment.

A patient who has run afoul of social standards or violated professional boundaries, whose fetish has been discovered, may have no motivation to change an otherwise pleasurable means of sexual gratification but may regret being discovered and work to prevent recurrence. The man who has been discovered by his employer while viewing images of nude men in new shoes, or the man charged with stealing women's underwear from a neighbor's dirty clothes hamper, may benefit from a focus on reducing the compulsive nature of the behavior that allowed it to slip beyond their control, treating compulsive sexual behavior or kleptomania. Alternatively the podiatrist who has come to attention for innocently asking a known patient to suck on her toes may have personality pathology or interpersonal dysfunction that precipitated the gross misjudgment of social propriety and neglect of professional ethics.

Treatment is not begun until a systematic developmental sexual history is completed. This process is part of a larger effort to understand the nonsexual developmental forces of the patient's life—i.e., his dynamics. When the physician has spent a considerable effort to understand the man's history, intellectual and social capacities, and private attitudes towards his fetish, a treatment process can begin.

A common mode of presentation derives from complaints about the psychological and sexual intimacies of a couple, with motivation to change in order to accommodate the partner. The most distressed person is usually the partner who has insisted upon getting professional assistance. As the history unfolds beyond a presenting complaint of low sexual desire, it emerges that both partners are angry at one another and that the relationship is in crisis. He, the fetishist, is feeling betrayed that after years of marriage she is now demanding that he desist with the behavior that she had until then permitted. The wife, seeking to deepen the intimacy of their marriage, is enraged and humiliated as she sees more clearly that she is not the source of his pleasure at all, and perhaps never has been.

Clinical Case Example

A couple with three grown emancipated children presented for help because of erectile dysfunction. Only on the third visit did the couple reveal that their lovemaking for 30 years was dependent upon a ritual. He insisted that they both put on full-length slips and lie in bed silently for a few minutes. He then would begin to caress her and quickly move to intercourse. When she insisted that she no longer could tolerate making love to a man who had to pretend she was an old lady, he asked whether he could at least hold the slip. When she refused even this compromise, he was unable to erect. On occasion, when she relented he was securely potent.

Goals of treatment in this or other cases of fetishistic disorder may include:

1. Decreasing the intensity of the fetishistic arousal
2. Increasing interest in normative sexual behavior, as negotiated with the partner
3. Decreasing shame associated with the erotic fixation
4. Preventing victimization or illegal activity
5. Improving romantic or other interpersonal disturbances that are pervasive in a patient's social or occupational life

Behavioral treatments have been attempted, utilizing a range of aversion techniques in addition to reconditioning to traditional erotic targets. Effectiveness of these treatments has been reported, but without evidence for sustained decreases in eroticization of a fetish [14]. Cognitive techniques of thought stopping, in combination with gradual and repeated introduction of more acceptable fantasies and behaviors may be utilized [15, 16], with success depending upon the motivation of the patient or couple, and the quality of the working therapeutic relationship. Traditional techniques to improve relationship dynamics, from teaching assertiveness and communication skills to education on patterns of sexual desire and arousal, or sensate focus exercises to target sexual functioning may all be a part of treatment.

Treatment of couples who present often involves helping both partners to understand the need for a fetish in developmental terms. Many of these men had significant discontinuities in their parental relationships. The man and his wife often benefit from an explanation that is beyond the verification of the behavioral sciences. The explanation is actually a hypothesis that gathers in the details of the man's development. For example, the fetish sometimes is a representation of the mother and functions just as a soft toy does for a toddler at bedtime, enabling self-soothing. It comforts him and distracts him from his anxiety about being an adequate man or his fears about a woman's dangerous body, and allows him to be excited. What explanations to share depends not only on the therapist's grasp of and belief in the childhood origins of fetishism but in the patient and the partner's capacity to make sense of the sexual limitations in terms of his past attachment and fears. Fetishistic disorder is not so much cured as managed by the couple over time with understanding, affection, and humor, and it may not matter what ideological form of explanation is offered.

Medication treatment may have a role in managing fetishistic disorder. Case studies have indicated some successes [17], but medications have not been subject to randomized controlled trials and are not FDA approved. Positive effects of serotonergic modulation have been reported, separately with fluoxetine and clomipramine [18, 19]. The effectiveness of these medications may utilize either the suppression of sexual functioning or the treatment of the obsessive fixation on an object seen in fetishistic disorder, given the similarities to obsessive compulsive disorder, though the latter theory remains untested. Anti-androgenic or anti-dopaminergic agents are also likely to have effect in global suppression of sexual functioning, including fetishistic behavior but also desire and drive. Risk profiles need to be discussed with the patient in addition to the perceived benefits of the asexual state, were this to be the patient's preference. Suppressive therapies should only be pursued if efforts in psychotherapy of normalization and acceptance, integration, and other behavioral change techniques have failed or are not options.

Opioid and oxytocin systems also hold promise in moderating fetishistic drive and increasing normosexual partnered activity, though evidence for this is largely absent. Naltrexone has been identified in several case studies as having positive effect in combination with psychotherapy at managing fetishistic disorder comorbid with substance use disorders [20].

Conclusion

Fetishistic disorder may be challenging to diagnose and difficult to treat, and the research base to guide these practices has not developed significantly. Mental health professionals have long observed the nuances of fetishism in the sexual lives of their patents, though modern research is yet to find the impetus to expand the evidence base on this subject. Fetishistic disorder has maintained its place in the DSM as well as in the popular imagination, due to a combination of fascination and prevalence of the condition, though the latter remains difficult to quantify. The vast growth in recent years of technologies to facilitate individual expression of sexual variance as well as subcultural intercommunication and allegiance have already played a role in normalizing sexual variation. The paraphilia of fetishism is high on the list of sexual variations that stand to develop further in upcoming years, both in the cultural landscape and the annals of evidence based medicine. These developments are likely to bring changes both to the diagnosis and management of fetishistic disorder, and to further enrich our clinical understanding of the sexual imagination.

References

1. Kafka M. The DSM, diagnostic criteria for fetishism. Arch Sex Behav. 2010;39:357.
2. American Psychiatric Association. Diagnostic and statistical manual of mental disorders (DSM-5). 5th ed. Arlington: American Psychiatric Association; 2013.

3. Hawkinson K, Zamboni B. Adult baby/diaper lovers: an exploratory study of an online community sample. Arch Sex Behav. 2014;43:863–77.
4. Abel GG, Osborn C. The paraphilias. The extent and nature of sexually deviant and criminal behavior. Psychiatr Clin North Am. 1992;15:675.
5. Blanchard R. The DSM, diagnostic criteria for transvestic fetishism. Arch Sex Behav. 2010;39:363.
6. Weinberg MS, Williams CJ, Calhan C. Homosexual foot fetishism. Arch Sex Behav. 1994;23:611.
7. Scorolli C, Ghirlanda S, Enquist M, et al. Relative prevalence of different fetishes. Int J Impot Res. 2007;19:432.
8. Nersessian E. A cat as fetish: a contribution to the theory of fetishism. Int J Psychoanal. 1998;79(Pt 4):713.
9. Mitchell W, Falconer M, Hill D. Epilepsy with fetishism relieved by temporal lobectomy. Lancet. 1954;267(6839):626–30.
10. Abel GG, Coffey L, Osborn CA. Sexual arousal patterns: normal and deviant. Psychiatr Clin North Am. 2008;31:643.
11. Martin SF, Levine SB. Fetishistic disorder. uptodate.com. Accessed October 23, 2016.
12. Stoller RJ. Perversion. New York: Random House; 1975. p. 132.
13. Freund K, Blanchard R. Erotic target location errors in male gender dysphorics, paedophiles, and fetishists. Br J Psychiatry. 1993;162:558.
14. Wise TN. Fetishism: etiology and treatment. A review from multiple perspectives. Compr Psychiatry. 1985;26:249.
15. Wiederman M. Paraphilia and fetishism. Family J. 2003;11:315.
16. Darcangelo S, Hollings A, Paladino G. Fetishism: assessment and treatment. In: Laws D, O'Donohue W, editors. Sexual deviance: theory, assessment and treatment. New York: Guilford; 2008.
17. Guay D. Drug treatment of paraphilic and nonparaphilic sexual disorders. Clin Ther. 2009;31:1.
18. Lorefice LS. Fluoxetine treatment of a fetish. J Clin Psychiatry. 1991;52:41.
19. Clayton AH. Fetishism and clomipramine. Am J Psychiatry. 1993;150:673.
20. Firoz K, Sankar V, Rajmohan V. Treatment of fetishism with naltrexone: a case report. Asian J Psychiatr. 2014;8:67.

Chapter 12
Transvestic Disorder

Richard Balon

The word "transvestism" generally means cross-dressing, regardless of its purpose. In popular language, it is also associated with acting in a manner or style associated with the other sex. In sexuology, the term transvestism, from the Latin "trans" (across, over) and "vestitus" (dress, and dressed, clothed) was introduced by Magnus Hirschfeld in 1910 in his book *The Transvestites: The erotic drive to cross dressing*. Though the term transvestism is just about a hundred years old, there have been references to transvestic behavior/cross-dressing in the Bible [1] and in the writings of Herodotus and Hippocrates. They described some Scythian males wearing female clothes, and ascribed their cross-dressing to depression (so-called Melancholia Scythorum). Some Roman Emperors, e.g., Caligula, Heliogabalus (aka Elagabalus, possibly transgendered) and Nero, cross-dressed [2].

R. Balon, M.D. (✉)
Department of Psychiatry and Behavioral Neurosciences, Wayne State University, Tolan Park Building, 3rd Floor, 3901 Chrysler Service Dr., Detroit, MI 48201, USA

Department of Anesthesiology, Wayne State University, Tolan Park Building, 3rd Floor, 3901 Chrysler Service Dr., Detroit, MI 48201, USA
e-mail: rbalon@wayne.edu

R. Balon (ed.), *Practical Guide to Paraphilia and Paraphilic Disorders*, DOI 10.1007/978-3-319-42650-1_12

Transvestism, in the narrow sense of sexuology and psychiatry, means deriving sexual arousal from cross-dressing. However, it seems that psychiatry has not always settled on what the term transvestism and transvestic disorder really encompasses, and what name or term we should use. The DSM-III [3] used the term transvestism, while DSM-III-R [4] introduced the term transvestic fetishism, which was also used in DSM-IV [5]. The DSM-5 [6] returned to using the term transvestism and introduced the distinction between transvestism and transvestic disorder (similar to other paraphilias/paraphilic disorders, see below). One of the DSM-5 specifiers (see below) denotes whether transvestism/transvestic disorder occurs with fetishism (being *specifically* sexually aroused by *fabrics, materials, or garments*).

Wheeler, Newring, and Draper ([7], p 273) pointed out that the term "transvestite" has been applied to various persons engaged in cross-dressing for different reasons than transvestism. These include individuals who are *transsexual* (a person dissatisfied with her/his biological sex and who wishes to live permanently as, and be perceived as, a person of opposite sex); *transgendered* (a person who is satisfied with her/his biological sex, but at some or all time prefers the social role or behavior typically associated with the other gender); *androgynous* (a person dissatisfied with her/his biological sex and gender role, but derives satisfaction from some cross-gender expression); *gender mimic* (a person satisfied with her/his biological sex and gender role but mimics or spoofs the opposite sex for entertainment or occupation—e.g., a man posing as a drag queen); or *effeminate homosexuals*. Some of the DSM editions included an exclusion criterion partially addressing this issue, e.g., that an individual with transvestism does not meet the criteria for transsexualism [3], or gender identity disorder of non-transsexual type, or transsexualism [4]. The important difference is that none of these cross-dressing individuals (transsexuals, transgendered, androgynous, gender mimic, or effeminate homosexuals) derives sexual arousal from cross-dressing. Thus, it is important to consider all these possibilities and variations when discussing the patient's cross-dressing.

Cross-dressing may also occur in the cultural and religious context, e.g., some male devotees of the Hindu God Krishna may dress in female clothes; in Italy in some processions in the street of Naples and other places femminielli (feminine males, or gay men) wear female wedding dresses. Hijras of South Asia are male-to-female transsexuals or transgendered persons dressed as females and recognized as a third gender by some governments (e.g., Bangladesh, Pakistan). Similar to this are the kathoyes of Thailand, or otokonokos of Japan. On the other hand, wearing a kilt or sarong does not necessarily mean cross-dressing, but rather a cultural custom or tradition.

Cross-dressing is definitely a complex issue with many layers related and unrelated to sexuality. Cross-dressing in terms of transvestism/transvestic disorder is just a part of this wide spectrum and is actually rare.

Diagnostic Criteria

The DSM-5 Criteria of transvestic disorder [5] are as follows (Reprinted with permission from the Diagnostic and Statistical Manual of Mental Disorders, Fifth Edition, (Copyright 2013). American Psychiatric Association.):

> *Criterion A: Over a period of at least 6 months, recurrent and intense sexual arousal from cross-dressing, as manifested by fantasies, urges, or behaviors.*
>
> *Criterion B: The fantasies, sexual urges, or behaviors cause clinically significant distress or impairment in social, occupational or other important areas of functioning.*
>
> *Specify if:*
>
> *With fetishism: if sexually aroused by fabrics, materials, or garments.*
>
> *With autogynephilia: If sexually aroused by thoughts or images of self as female.*
>
> *Specify:*
>
> *In controlled environment: This specifier is primarily applicable to individuals living in institutional or other settings where opportunities to engage in voyeuristic behavior are restricted.*
>
> *In full remission: The individual has not acted on the urges with a nonconsenting person, and there has been no distress or impairment in social, occupational or other areas of functioning, for at least 5 years while in an uncontrolled environment.*

As noted before, the existence of sexual arousal derived from cross-dressing has been the central point in making the diagnosis of transvestism/transvestic disorder. In males (transvestism is extremely rare in females), sexual arousal in a form of erection may co-occur with cross-dressing in various forms—young male may masturbate and remove female clothing, older males may avoid penis stimulation to prolong the cross-dressing session [6]. Interestingly, the lack of cross-dressing during the intercourse with a female partner may lead to difficulties to maintain erection during the intercourse [6].

The diagnostic criteria of transvestism have changed over time, being influenced by new observations and thinking. The DSM-III [3] criteria emphasized the frustration when cross-dressing was interfered with, and the person with this paraphilia should not meet diagnostic criteria for transexualism. DSM-III-R [4] added gender identity disorder to the exclusion criteria, and similar exclusion (gender dysphoria) was kept in DSM-IV [5], while exclusionary criterion of transsexualism was not. The disorder was still called transvestic fetishism [5]. Blanchard ([8], p 365) noted that the use of the diagnostic term of transvestic fetishism was probably an attempt to "disambiguate the term *transvestism*, which was then, as now, sometimes used to denote cross-dressing homosexual men ("drag queens"), and which had historically also been used to denote transsexuals." Blanchard [8] also felt that the "the name choice of *Transvestic Fetishism* was counterheuristic. It stresses one frequent feature of transvestism (erotic interest in the material properties of women's clothing) at the expense of another one (erotic arousal at the thought or image of oneself as woman)." Blanchard [8] then proposed diagnostic criteria that are almost identical with the DSM-5 criteria. However, for the first time, the DSM-5 [6] criteria make for the diagnosis of transvestism/transvestic disorder gender neutral—it does not specify that this behavior has to occur in a heterosexual male. It also removes fetishism from the name of this paraphilia/paraphilic disorder and moves it to one of its specifiers.

The first specifier, *with fetishism*, denotes only fabrics, materials, or garments as sexually arousing fetishes, in contrast to fetishism/fetishistic disorder, which notes the role of using nonliving objects or a highly specific focus on nongenital body part(s) in deriving sexual arousal (and emphasizes that it should not be limited to articles of clothing used in cross-dressing). The second specifier, *with autogynephilia*, notes sexual arousal due to thoughts or images of self as female, or, as Blanchard writes [8–10] a male propensity to be erotically aroused by the thought or image of himself as a female. According to some (e.g., [11, 12]) autogynephilia is the paraphilia that underlies all, or almost all, cases of male transvestism and many cases of male-to-female transexualism ([12], p 135). Lawrence [12] suggested that it is a surprisingly prevalent condition that is not widely recognized or understood, and it is underappreciated by clinicians. According to DSM-5 ([6], p 703), autogynephilic fantasies may focus on exhibiting female physiological functions (e.g., lactation), stereotypical feminine behavior (e.g., knitting), or on possessing female anatomy.

The diagnostic considerations need to carefully parse the underlying reasons for cross-dressing. As Wheeler, Newring, and Draper [7] and Docter and Prince [13] noted, there are subgroups of transvestites. One group could be called "nuclear transvestites." Those are psychologically satisfied with their gender and sexual identity as males; they are stable periodic cross-dressers [13]. The second group could be called "marginal transvestites." They are not satisfied with their gender and sexual identity as males, and may desire additional means of feminization (hormones, etc.) [7, 13]. These "marginal transvestites" may include persons who identify themselves as transgendered or transsexuals, and who engage in cross-dressing for more than sexual gratification [7].

Summary of Evidence

The prevalence of transvestism/transvestic disorder is considered to be low. The question is what low really means. The DSM-5 [6] notes that less than 3 % of males reported having ever being sexually aroused by cross-dressing. Langstrom and Zucker [14] in a random sample of 2450 persons 18–60 years old in Sweden reported that 2.8 % of men and 0.4 % of women admitted to at least one episode of transvestic fetishism.

The age of onset of transvestism/transvestic disorder is a bit complicated to determine and thus not much is known about it. The DSM-5 [6] suggests that the first sign of transvestism may occur during childhood as fascination with a particular item of female clothing or female clothing in general. As Wheeler, Newring, and Draper ([7], p 278) point out, at this stage children may experience cross-dressing as pleasurable and exciting in a more generalized, rather than a sexual way. However, the limited way we have been able to study transvestism/transvestic disorder, especially its course, cannot confirm this explanation beyond speculations. The survey studies of persons with transvestism were of retrospective character, relying on patients' memories. We also do not know the frequency of pleasurable (non-sexual!) cross-dressing during childhood of persons who did not develop transvestism/transvestic disorder. Puberty seems to be the developmental period when cross-dressing begins to elicit sexual arousal and may, in some cases, lead to ejaculation [6].

Similarly, the information about the course of transvestism/transvestic disorder is based on very little solid information. The course may be continuous or episodic. The peak of transvestic interests and behavior is during early adulthood. In some individuals the sexual excitement brought by cross-dressing gradually decreases and may be replaced by feeling of comfort and well-being [6]. It seems that the frequency of cross-dressing decreases with increasing age. Some transvestites may progress to gender dysphoria as they become more and more interested in their female role [6]. Interestingly, in the study by Langstrom and Zucker [14], more than 50 % of those reporting sexual arousal from cross-dressing did not see it as acceptable to self, their sexual practice was ego-dystonic.

Some studies focused on various characteristics of persons with transvestism or transvestic fetishism. In a study by Docter and Prince [13] cross-dressers described themselves mostly as heterosexuals (87 %) and most of them had ever married (83 %, and actually 60 % at the time of the study). Langstrom and Zucker [14] reported that separation from parents, same-sex sexual experiences, being easily sexually aroused (either due to higher arousability or lower control of sexual impulses), pornography use, and higher masturbation frequency were significantly associated with transvestic fetishism. They also found that transvestic fetishism was "strongly associated with ever having been sexually aroused from using pain when having sex, having exposed one's genitalia to a stranger, and spying on what others are doing sexually" ([14], p 94). Langstrom and Zucker found this a bit worrisome as these are proxy measures of paraphilias/parahilic disorders with the possibility to harm others. Transvestic fetishism or transvestism may be also associated with sexual risk of acting out [14]. In general, transvestism/transvestic disorder seems to be associated with hypersexuality. There has not been much focus on wives/partners of persons with transvestism/transvestic disorder. Most women (83 %) in the study by Docter and Prince [13] were aware of their husband's transvestism, though only one-third were informed before marriage. About 19 % were "completely antagonistic," 28 % were "completely accepting," of their husband's behavior, and the rest was less clear about it.

There are various theories of the etiology of transvestism/transvestic behavior. Many of them propose various psychogenic origins, such as behavioral and reinforcement theory akin to classical conditioning (pairing accidental exposure to female clothing with a pleasurable experience), family-origin considerations (e.g., family constellation and parental relationships—[15]), impact of sexual abuse in childhood, and psychoanalytical explanation (mostly based in castration anxiety). In 1965, Housden [16] reviewed the literature for evidence of biological etiology of transvestism and found no evidence for it. The state of knowledge and opinion about the biological etiology of transvestism remains the same 50 years later. It is important to note that the efficacy of some biological treatments (antidepressants, hormones) in transvestism does not prove biological etiology, as the effects of treatments are nonspecific, similar to other paraphilias/paraphilic disorders.

The most important part of the assessment of a person with transvestism/transvestic disorder is a thorough clinical interview. The discussion of present illness should focus on a careful description of cross-dressing and its relationship to sexual arousal. The lack of sexual arousal during cross-dressing suggests the absence of transvestism and possible presence of other issues such as transsexualism, transgenderism, or gender dysphoria. The existence and degree of distress and/or impairment *due* to cross-dressing needs to be also established. The history should include past psychiatric history, medical history, family history, careful psychosexual and developmental history, history of possible substance abuse, social and relationship history, educational/occupational history and history of criminal behavior or legal problems. The sexual history should pay special attention to any sexual dysfunction, onset of transvestic behavior and its course, existence of other paraphilic tendencies/behaviors and overlap with other paraphilias/paraphilic disorders, history of sexual acting out or sexual violence, and association of substance abuse with episodes of cross-dressing. A useful part of the initial evaluation could be an interview with collateral sources (e.g., partner, spouse), including obtaining information about the impact of transvestism on relationships.

There are no specific diagnostic tests for transvestism/transvestic disorder. At times, useful information can be obtained from intelligence testing, or from the personality profile (using the MMPI or Millon Clinical Multiaxial Inventory). The usefulness of physiological measures such as phallometric assessment in the diagnosis of transvestism/transvestic disorder has not been established.

Information about treatment of transvestism/transvestic disorder is again scarce. In contrast to most other paraphilias/paraphilic disorders we do not have treatment information from prison-based or other legally mandated treatment programs, as transvestism/transvestic disorder is generally not considered criminal behavior [17]. Usually, only a few true transvestites look for treatment (though in a study by Docter and Prince [13] 45 % subjects reported consulting with either a psychiatrist or a psychologist and 67 % of them reported that they gained some benefit).

Other issues that may explain the lack of information about treatment of transvestism/transvestic disorder are: (a) the change of the name (transvestism vs. transvestic fetishism) within our diagnostic systems over the years, and (b) the perceived or real overlap with other entities possibly involving cross-dressing, such as transsexualism and transgenderism. For instance, there are more self-help books and self-help groups available for individuals with transgender or transsexual issues than for persons suffering from transvestism/transvestic disorder (almost none). The mostly case report based literature on pharmacotherapy (summarized by Newring, Wheeler and Draper—[17]) is also a bit confusing, as some cases describe transvestic fetishism, some transvestism, some fetishism, and some an overlap of various paraphilic behaviors.

Last but not least is the issue of cross-dressing vs. distress. The literature usually includes cases describing treatment successful in decreasing transvestic behavior, or fantasies and urges. However, it is conceivable that at least some persons with transvestism/transvestic disorder seek treatment which would mainly focus on alleviating their distress. The distress over cross-dressing or over social or other impairment due to cross-dressing may be alleviated in therapy or by some medications, yet cross-dressing and sexual arousal may continue. We simply do not know whether this is happening and is not reported in the literature.

Newring, Wheeler, and Draper [17] recommend various therapy approaches, such as relapse prevention, harm reduction, dialectical behavior therapy, and functional analytic psychotherapy (which focuses also on interpersonal nature of the patient's life). However, these recommendations are not evidence-based and not even supported by solid case reports. There is one case report from Taiwan [18] describing the use of cognitive-behavioral therapy and supportive therapy in an adolescent transvestic fetishist. He was able to stop his behavior and had fewer sexually arousing fantasies after 18 psychotherapy sessions over more than 4 months.

Newring, Wheeler, and Draper [17] also suggest self-help and support societies.

Most of the reports of pharmacological treatment of transvestism/transvestic disorder (or previously transvestic fetishism) involve serotonergic medications such as SSRIs and buspirone. There are only a few cases of pharmacotherapy of true transvestism or transvestic fetishism. Fedoroff published two independent cases [19, 20] of successful treatment of transvestic fetishism with buspirone, a serotonergic anxiolytic. The first case is especially interesting: the patient, a 46-year-old married man reported decrease of transvestic fetishism urges in 9 days and stopped cross-dressing in 3 weeks. He stopped his treatment after 3 months, but his urges came back. He was restarted on buspirone 15 mg/day and improved again. The second case [20] involved a patient with atypical paraphilia and transvestic fetishism responding to buspirone.

Usmani and colleagues [21] described a case of a 17-year-old Indian man presenting with a desire to wear his mother clothes, wearing them and masturbating while dressed in them. He improved on fluoxetine 40 mg/day. Ward [22] administered lithium to a 24-year-old manic-depressive man with transvestism. Transvestic behavior disappeared shortly after lithium was started. Brantley and Wise [23] successfully used diethylstilbestrol to reduce the desire to cross-dress in a 65-year-old gender-dysphoric transvestite. These two cases are complicated by comorbidity and thus it is difficult to fully appreciate the effect of treatment on transvestism. In an interesting case, Riley [24] observed a 72-year-old man with a long history of Parkinson's disease who developed cross-dressing and hypersexuality after being treated with selegiline. The symptomatology ceased after selegiline was discontinued. Most other cases cited in the literature and reviewed by Newring, Wheeler, and Draper [17] are cases of fetishism or of multiple paraphilias, not really of transvestism.

Clinical Example (Fictitious Case Combining Features of Several Cases)

A 30-year-old single man computer analyst came to "get help with my so called problem behavior." He states that as long as he can remember, he has loved to dress in female clothes, especially in female underwear. Cross-dressing sexually excites him, he gets an erection and occasionally ejaculates. He has been comfortable with his male gender and sexuality, though he has "wondered at times how it is to be a woman, what the female sexual experience is, what they feel differently." He never considered his behavior problematic. He has been able to maintain regular sexual relationships with several girlfriends, "though wearing female clothes was more arousing at times." Some of his girlfriends knew about his transvestism and tolerated it.

He says that as he has been "carelessly" walking around in female clothes, thus some of his neighbors noticed it. He lives in a close-knit suburban community and rumors about his cross-dressing quickly spread around the neighborhood. Some kids called him a "queer" while he was jogging in a neighborhood park. Several adults from the neighborhood asked him whether he was "a deviant, because we do not want deviants around our kids." Finally, the rumors reached his employer, who questioned him about his rumored cross-dressing and worrying about "the company's reputation."

He has gradually become anxious and mildly depressed, worrying about his job and safety. He was upset because "how can they ask about my sexual preferences, I have not harmed or endangered anyone!" His performance at work deteriorated, as he was not able to fully concentrate on his tasks. He said he needed to "put myself together" to be able to work as well as he used to, prior to being questioned about his behavior. He was more worried about his job performance and anxiety than about his cross-dressing, as "that is what I really enjoy."

He agreed to start cognitive-behavioral therapy and to try buspirone, starting dose 10 mg/day with gradual increase to

30 mg/day. However, he called to cancel his next appointment in about 2 weeks. He stated that though he has been starting to feel better and having fewer urges to cross-dress, "I cannot live in this intolerant community and work for my employer, I am leaving town, I found a job in New York. People there are more tolerant and one is more anonymous there."

Recommendations

Transvestism/transvestic disorder is a relatively "popular or popularized," paraphilia. However, as defined in the narrow terms of our classification systems, it is relatively rare and not many persons seek treatment for this condition.

The evaluation of a person seeking help should start with a detailed clinical interview conducted in a comfortable and trusting environment. Special attention should be paid to the possibility of other coexisting paraphilias and/or transsexualism, transgender issues, and gender mimic. The presence of sexually arousing cross-dressing needs to be established for making correct diagnosis. Patients should be also asked about possible sexual fetishes and about being aroused by images of himself being a female (autogynephilia). Distress and impairment in various areas of functioning should be explored and it should be established what the distress is really about ("my behavior" vs. reaction of the environment). Collateral information from partner/family should be obtained, if possible.

The goals of treatment (decrease of cross-dressing, decrease of distress) should be established and discussed with the patient. Treatment should start with psychotherapy. No transvestism specific psychotherapy has really been established as effective in the treatment of transvestism/transvestic disorder. Supportive therapy and CBT should probably be initiated first. Functional analytic psychotherapy or dialectical behavioral therapy may also be introduced. Serotonergic medication such as buspirone and SSRIs may be helpful in reducing cross-dressing behavior and associated sexual arousal, and also with accompanying secondary symptomatology such as anxiety and depression. Buspirone may be the initial pharmacotherapy of choice due to its tolerability, but the evidence of its efficacy is fairly limited. Hormones such as antiandrogens should be reserved only for most extreme cases, including sexual violence or overlap with other paraphilias/paraphilic disorders. Treatment risks and side effects should always be discussed with the patient. Combining pharmacotherapy and psychotherapy seems prudent, though there is no evidence addressing treatment combinations.

Comprehensive treatment should also include a referral to self-help groups. Contact for *Tri-Ess Crossdressers—The Society for the Second Self: An international social and support group for heterosexual crossdressers, their partners, the spouses of married cross-dressers, and their families* could be found online. Unfortunately, self-help books devoted solely to transvestism/transvestic disorder are not available. However, psychoeducation about parahilias/paraphilic disorders by the treating clinician could be helpful. Finally, whenever possible, the patient's partner/spouse should be included in the treatment and joint sessions may be helpful.

References

1. Aggrawal A. References to the paraphilias and sexual crimes in the Bible. J Forensic Leg Med. 2009;16:109–14.
2. Brierley H. Transvestism: a handbook with case studies for psychologists, psychiatrists and counselors. New York: Pergamon Press; 1979.
3. American Psychiatric Association. Diagnostic and statistical manual of mental disorders. 3rd ed. Washington, DC: American Psychiatric Association; 1980.
4. American Psychiatric Association. Diagnostic and statistical manual of mental disorders. 3rd ed., rev. Washington, DC: American Psychiatric Association; 1987.
5. American Psychiatric Association. Diagnostic and statistical manual of mental disorders. 4th ed. Washington, DC: American Psychiatric Association; 1994.

6. American Psychiatric Association. Diagnostic and statistical manual of mental disorders. 5th ed. Arlington: American Psychiatric Association; 2013. p. 702–4.
7. Wheeler J, Newring KAB, Draper C. Transvestic fetishism. Psychopathology and theory. In: Laws DR, O'Donohue WT, editors. Sexual deviance. Theory, assessment, and treatment. 2nd ed. New York: Guilford; 2008. p. 272–84.
8. Blanchard R. The diagnostic criteria for transvestic fetishism. Arch Sex Behav. 2019;39:363–72.
9. Blanchard R. The classification and labeling of nonhomosexual gender dysphorias. Arch Sex Behav. 1989;18:315–34.
10. Blanchard R. The concept of autogynephilia and the typology of male gender dysphoria. J Nerv Ment Dis. 1989;177:616–23.
11. Blanchard R. Clinical observations and systematic studies of autogynephilia. J Sex Marital Ther. 1991;17:235–51.
12. Lawrence A. Autogynephilia: an underappreciated paraphilia. In: Balon R, editor. Sexual dysfunction: beyond the brain-body connection. Basel: Larger AG; 2011. p. 135–48.
13. Docter RF, Prince V. Transvestism: a survey of 1032 cross-dressers. Arch Sex Behav. 1997;26:589–605.
14. Langstrom N, Zucker KJ. Transvestic fetishism in the general population: prevalence and correlates. J Sex Marital Ther. 2005;31:87–95.
15. Schott RL. The childhood and family dynamics of transvestites. Arch Sex Behav. 1995;24:309–26.
16. Housden J. An examination of the biological etiology of transvestism. Int J Soc Psychiatry. 1965;11:301–5.
17. Newring KAB, Wheeler J, Draper C. Transvestic fetishism. Assessment and treatment. In: Laws DR, O'Donohue WT, editors. Sexual deviance. Theory, assessment, and treatment. 2nd ed. New York: Guilford; 2008. p. 285–304.
18. Chiang YL, Yeh SS, Hsiao CC, Ree SC. Treatment of a transvestic fetishist with cognitive-behavioral therapy and supportive therapy. Changgeng Yi Xue Za Zhi. 1999;22:299–312.
19. Fedoroff JP. Buspirone hydrochloride in the treatment of transvestic fetishism. J Clin Psychiatry. 1988;49:408–9.
20. Fedoroff JP. Buspirone hydrochloride in the treatment of an atypical paraphilia. Arch Sex Behav. 1992;21:401–6.
21. Usmani MA, Gaur RK, Azmi SA, Gangwar S. Treatment of transvestic fetishism with fluoxetine: a case report. Iran J Psychiatry Behav Sci. 2012;6:100–1.

22. Ward NG. Successful lithium treatment of transvestism associated with manic-depression. J Nerv Ment Dis. 1975;161:204–6.
23. Brantley JT, Wise TH. Antiandrogenic treatment of a gender-dysphoric transvestite. J Sex Marital Ther. 1985;11:109–12.
24. Riley DE. Reversible transvestic fetishism in a man with Parkinson's disease treated with selegiline. Clin Neuropharmacol. 2002;25:234–7.

Chapter 13
Other Specified Paraphilic Disorders

Peer Briken, Verena Klein, and Fritjof von Franqué

Introduction

Sexuality as a clinical research topic, the question of what is to be regarded as normality, variation, as a problem or a disorder, cannot be stable over time and not be understood without its cultural embeddedness. Medical science defines sexual disorders, inter alia on the levels of deviations, functional limitations, suffering, and danger to others in a reciprocal relationship between society and the individual. During the last years we learned from research that previously called "unusual" sexual fantasies are commonly found [1].

During sexual fantasies violations of borders are common in active as well as in passive forms. Fortunately, it is less common that people violate the borders of others through sexual offences. It also succeeds that clinical sex research distinguishes better between sexual desires and actions nowadays. For example, sadomasochistic sexuality (e.g., BDSM practices; see Chapter xxx in this book) can be distinguished from forced sexual acts [2] and a sexual interest in children from

P. Briken, M.D., F.E.C.S.M. (✉) • V. Klein, Dipl.-Psych.
F. von Franqué, Dipl.-Psych., ECPS
Institute for Sex Research and Forensic Psychiatry, University Medical Centre Hamburg-Eppendorf, Martinistr. 52, Hamburg 20255, Germany
e-mail: briken@uke.de; vklein@uke.de; f.von-franque@uke.de

R. Balon (ed.), *Practical Guide to Paraphilia and Paraphilic Disorders*, DOI 10.1007/978-3-319-42650-1_13

child abuse [3]. Antisocial and psychopathic traits might even pose a more significant risk for sexual offenses than the paraphilic interests (e.g., [4]). Especially when accompanied by antisocial personality traits the line between fantasy and reality sometimes is very narrow and permeable for externalized aggressive desires. Unfortunately, experiences that people are violated sexually are and will be a social reality.

Among the "other paraphilias" phenomena such as obscene telephone calls, necrophilia, coprophilia, klismaphilia, zoophilia, and urolagnia are subsumed as well as strangulation and autoasphyxia to increase sexual excitement, a preference for partners with anatomical abnormalities (such as amputated limbs), and many other sexual arousal patterns that seem unusual or meaningless for many people. Both clinical and everyday forensic psychiatric practitioners have rather less to do with these disorders. Nevertheless, at least some of these may be less often than most people realize. However, many people that are aroused by such sexual stimuli feel ashamed and do not seek help. Or they never acted out their interest against a non-consenting individual and do only suffer from the social rejection accompanied by their interest but not from the arousal pattern itself. Some of these individuals in a more narrow sense do not fulfill the criteria of a paraphilic disorder but can still profit from counseling. Others do not need any help at all.

Today, it is much easier to live with a special sexual interest like coprophilia or urolagnia because of an easier access to specific pornography and the possibility to arrange sexual contacts or partners with similar inclinations via digital media. The existing market for pornography simultaneously suggests that at least there is a significant number of people who is interested in corresponding material.

Diagnostic Criteria and Assessment Process

The category of other paraphilic disorders applies to patients in which a recurrent and intense sexual arousal or behavior that does not meet the full criteria for any of the specific paraphilic disorders but causes clinically significant distress or impairment in social, occupational, or other important areas of functioning. Examples of forms that can be specified include *telephone scatologia* (sexually aroused by obscene phone calls), *necrophilia* (sexually aroused by corpses), *zoophilia* (sexually aroused by animals), *coprophilia* (sexually arousal by feces), *klismaphilia* (sexually aroused by enemas), or *urophilia* (sexually aroused by urine) that has been present for at least 6 months and causes marked distress or impairment in social, occupational, or other important areas of functioning. In the DSM-5 [5] these disorders can be specified as "in remission" or as occurring "in a controlled environment."

Especially for this diagnostic category there is a substantial risk of an irrational extension to all possible, supposedly unusual sexual preferences, which are extremely rare in clinical practice. The usefulness of separate nosological categories for every single interest must therefore be questioned.

Table 13.1 shows the most important "other paraphilias." However, numerous other rare paraphilic interests have been described [6] like vampirism (erotic focus: blood), somnophilia (erotic focus: sleeping partner), hypoxyphilia (erotic focus: reduced oxygen intake), or gerontophilia (erotic focus: elderly partner). Many individuals presenting with such an interest do not fulfill the disorder (B)-criterion for a paraphilic disorder.

In a clinical context the "other paraphilias" are often presented in combination with the specific ones or in the context of sexual offending behavior. Especially in the combination with exhibitionism and/or voyeurism telephone scatologia may be understood as a form of courtship disorder [7] associated by relationship problems ([8]; see also the Case example below). In necrophilia the use of a corpse can be understood as a fetish-form of an unresisting or unrejecting partner. A central motive can be dominance, and necrophilia can be combined with forensic relevant sexual sadism causing a significant risk—sometimes also for sexual homicide [9]. In zoophilia individuals report to be drawn to animals out of a desire for affection but some people treat animals like sex objects without emotional attachment [10]. In our clinical forensic

Table 13.1 Examples of the other paraphilic disorders (Reprinted with permission from the Diagnostic and Statistical Manual of Mental Disorders, Fifth Edition, (Copyright 2013). American Psychiatric Association.)

Paraphilia	**Description**	**Frequent comorbidity with other paraphilias or specific forms of sexual offending**
Criterion A	Recurrent and intense sexual arousal (fantasies, urges and behaviors) involving…	
Telephone scatologia	Obscene telephone calls to unsuspecting victims	Exhibitionism Voyeurism
Necrophilia	A corpse	Sadism Cannibalism Sexual homicide
Zoophilia	Animals (mostly dogs or horses)	
Coprophilia	Feces	Sadomasochism
Klismaphilia	Enemas	Sadomasochism
Urophilia	Urine	Sadomasochism
Criterion B	The paraphilia has been present for at least 6 months and causes marked distress or impairment in social, occupational, or other important areas of functioning	

context zoophilic individuals often show social anxiety or schizoid personality characteristics. Some individuals that also share sadomasochistic sexual interests report coprophilic, klismaphilic, and urophilic interests.

Important issues in taking the sexual history in patients presenting with "other paraphilic disorders" include the development and content of sexual arousal and behavior patterns (age of onset, frequency and masturbation practice, sexual fantasies in childhood, adolescence and adulthood); the fantasies, desires, impulses and behavior within and beyond the partnership; the types and forms of pornography consumption (including the use of specific pornography presenting the paraphilic behavior or stimulus); paraphilic activities with prostitutes; experience of sexual and/or other violent assaults; sexual and general delinquency—criminal prosecutions.

For evaluation also specific questionnaires like the Multiphasic Sex Inventory [11] may be used. This instrument is an extensive true–false, self-report questionnaire consisting of statements about sexual activities, problems, and experiences. It is primarily intended to be used in assessing sexual offenders. It includes a variety of scales that also cover behaviors and fantasies associated with other paraphilic disorders.

Comorbidity with psychiatric disorders, esp. with mood disorders like depression, anxiety disorders, psychoactive substance abuse disorders, and personality disorders (antisocial, psychopathy, schizoid) should be evaluated. Since sexual fantasies and behaviors can be a form of coping with negative emotions or mood states that are related with the psychiatric conditions, it is necessary to start treatment planning with a thorough psychiatric diagnostic assessment.

If there is a risk for harm to others also a standardized prognostic assessment should be one of the first steps before developing a treatment plan. Risk assessment instruments like the Static-99 [12], the Stable-2007 [13], and the Sexual Violence Risk Scale [14] are useful measuring risk.

Summary of Evidence

The evidence for estimations of the prevalence, etiology, and risk caused by the "other paraphilic disorders" is weak. This is demonstrated through the low number of scientific publications. In MEDLINE (December 2015) the number of listed publications were as follows: telephone scatologia ($n=6$), necrophilia ($n=44$), zoophilia ($n=26$), coprophilia ($n=6$), klismaphilia ($n=6$), and urophilia ($n=2$).

To our knowledge there are no evidence based and well evaluated specific treatment programs for the "other paraphilic disorders." If there is a risk of danger to others, principles should guide treatment that have been established with sexual offenders with paraphilic interests [15–17]. If patients suffer from the symptoms themselves, the reduction of distress should be the primary treatment target. In some patients it is about both. Described are mainly cognitive-behavioral but also psychodynamic therapies and medical treatments [17]. To our knowledge special group therapy programs have not been offered because of the small number of cases in these rare disorders. Therapy is offered so far heavily customized in an individual setting. Therapy is often long lasting and must be sustained over the long term when there is a continuing risk of danger to others. In the background we find often complex comorbidities with personality disorders (e.g., schizoid example) or organic brain abnormalities. But also social anxiety and depression play a significant role.

Clinical Example

Mr A. was impaired by epilepsy since early childhood. While his brother was often punished and beaten by the father both parents treated Mr A. concerned about and controlling, barely trusted him to develop autonomy. From adolescence he was strongly inhibited in the contact with girls of his age. He never built a sexual relationship with a woman even later in adulthood. In late adolescence he committed a first sexual assault against a 13-year-old girl. He sexually fantasized about torturing girls or young women by administering enemas to them (of interest in this context is that it happened once in childhood that Mr A. received the administration of enemas while staying in hospital).

After the first consultation Mr. A. initially was treated with individual psychotherapy and medication with the GnRH-agonist leuprolide. The paraphilic symptoms showed a significant decline. However, the patient was no longer willing to take the medication after about a year because of erectile dysfunction that made masturbation for him almost impossible. Mr. A. was taken at this time in a group therapy treatment program and medication was switched to a selective serontonin reuptake inhibitor (fluoxetine 40 mg).

As it turned out later, at this point of treatment he started obscene phone calls for the first time in his life. He searched phone numbers from the phone book at random, asked girls or women that he wanted to give them an enema and tried to scare them by using obscene language while he masturbated. He often spent several hours with such calls and masturbated up to four times a day. Finally, the police determined Mr. A. The reason for the calls, Mr A. stated later, was that he found the calls less dangerous for him and others than fulfilling his fantasies in a direct, coercive contact with a child or a young women.

Mr. A. was sentenced to pay a fine and mandated for the continuation of treatment. He voluntarily agreed to a testosterone lowering therapy with cyproterone. He continued to be treated with psychotherapy in an individual setting. After several years of treatment with 50 mg initially and later 25 mg cyproterone medication was switched to an SSRI. Mr. A. is currently treated with an SSRI and still receives a low frequency relapse prevention oriented supportive psychotherapy. A relapse with obscene phone calls occurred in the meantime twice—but only in the short term. The patient admitted each one quickly. Hands on offenses did not occur.

Recommendations and Conclusions

To our knowledge there are no evidence based and well evaluated specific treatment programs for "the other paraphilic disorders" [17]. As with the specific paraphilias the primary goals for therapy are (1) the reduction of distress or impairment (if existent) via reducing fear of rejection or developing alternative forms of sexuality; and (2) the reduction of a possible risk for sexual offending (if existing) by a decrease in paraphilic sexual arousal, reducing sexual impulsivity and/or sexual preoccupation and improving sexual self-control. There is an ongoing debate regarding the possibility of changing the paraphilic interest itself. From an empirical point of view, this issue is still open to debate [22]. Clinically, patients report changes as well as very fixed paraphilic interests across the lifespan. Treatment providers should focus on individual cases in order to decide whether changes of paraphilic interests may be a realistic treatment goal.

Interventions to reduce associated mental health problems like social anxiety or depression and to change social skills can be helpful.

In the context of risk reduction, which most often leads to treatment in individuals with other paraphilic disorders the most influential theory is the Risk-Need-Responsivity (RNR-) model [18]. This model suggests that in an effective therapy:

- The intensity of treatment has to consider the risk potential for committing an offense (the higher the risk the more intensive therapy should be)
- The specific criminogenic needs like the paraphilic disorders should be particular therapy-goals
- Therapeutic programs should be used to which the specific individual can respond

These factors form the basis for psychotherapy as well as for medical treatment with SSRI, cyproterone, medroxprogesterone, and GnRH agonists. The decision for a pharmacological treatment is also depending on the severity of symptoms and risk [19–21]. For the evaluation of treatment success the abovementioned dynamic risk assessment instruments can be used.

References

1. Joyal CC, Cossette A, Lapierre V. What exactly is an unusual sexual fantasy? J Sex Med. 2015;12(2):328–40.
2. Martin SM, Smith F, Quirk SW. Discriminating coercive from sadomasochistic sexuality. Arch Sex Behav. 2016;45(5):1173–83. doi:10.1007/s10508-015-05950-0.
3. Dombert B, Schmidt AF, Banse R, Briken P, Hoyer J, Neutze J, Osterheider M. How common is men's self-reported sexual interest in prepubescent children? J Sex Res. 2015;4:1–10.

4. Klein V, Schmidt AF, Turner D, Briken P. Are sex drive and hypersexuality associated with pedophilic interest and child sexual abuse in a male community sample? PLoS One. 2015;10(7), e0129730.
5. American Psychiatric Association (APA). Diagnostisches und statistisches manual psychischer störungen DSM-5®. Göttingen: Hogrefe; 2015.
6. Milner JS, Dopke CA, Crouch JL. Paraphilia not otherwise specified. Psychopathology and theory. In: Laws RD, O'Donohue WT, editors. Sexual deviance. Theory, assessment, and treatment. 2nd ed. New York: Guilford; 2008. p. 384–418.
7. Freund K, Blanchard R. The concept of courtship disorder. J Sex Marital Ther. 1986;12:79–92.
8. Briken P, Nika E, Hill A, Berner W. Obszöne Telefonanrufe—Beziehungen zu Paraphilien, Paraphilie verwandten Störungen und "Stalking". Psychiatr Prax. 2005;32(6):304–7.
9. Briken P, Bourget D, Dufour M. Sexual sadism in sexual offenders and sexually motivated homicide. Psychiatr Clin North Am. 2014;37(2):215–30.
10. Kafka MP. The DSM, diagnostic criteria for paraphilia not otherwise specified. Arch Sex Behav. 2010;39(2):373–6.
11. Nichols HR, Molinder I. MSI—multiphasic sex inventory. Tacoma: Authors; 1984.
12. Hanson RK, Thornton D. Static 99: improving actuarial risk assessment for sex offenders. Ottawa: Department of the Solicitor General of Canada; 1999.
13. Hanson RK, Harris AJ, Scott TL, Helmus, L. Assessing the risk of sexual offenders on community supervision: The Dynamic Supervision Project; 2007. http://www.publicsafety.gc.ca/res/cor/rep/_fl/crp2007-05-en.pdf. Accessed 19 Aug 2010.
14. Boer DP, Hart SD, Kropp PR, Webster CD. Manual for the sexual violence risk. Burnaby: Simon Fraser University; 1997.
15. Hanson RK, Bourgon G, Helmus L, Hodgson S. The principles of effective correctional treatment also apply to sexual offenders. A meta-analysis. Crim Justice Behav. 2009;36:865–91.
16. Hanson RK, Yates PM. Psychological treatment of sex offenders. Curr Psychiatry Rep. 2013;15(3):348.
17. Penix TM. Paraphilia not otherwise specified. Assessment and treatment. In: Laws RD, O'Donohue WT, editors. Sexual deviance. Theory, assessment, and treatment. 2nd ed. New York: Guilford; 2008. p. 419–38.
18. Andrews DA, Bonta J. The psychology of criminal conduct. 5th ed. New Providence: LexisNexis Matthew Bender; 2010.

19. Briken P, Hill A, Berner W. Pharmacotherapy of paraphilias with long-acting agonists of luteinizing hormone-releasing hormone: a systematic review. J Clin Psychiatry. 2003;64:890–7.
20. Briken P, Hill A, Berner W. Pharmacotherapy of sexual offenders and men who are at risk of sexual offending. In: Boer D, Eher R, Miner MH, Pfäfflin F, Craig L, editors. International perspectives on the assessment and treatment of sexual offenders: theory, practice and research. Chichester: Wiley; 2011. p. 419–31.
21. Thibaut F, De La Barra F, Gordon H, Cosyns P, Bradford JMW, the WFSBP Task Force on Sexual Disorders. The world federation of Societies of Biological Psychiatry (WFSBP) Guidelines for the biological treatment of paraphilias. World J Biol Psychiatry. 2010;11:604–55.
22. Tozdan S, Briken P. 'I believed I could, so I did'—a theoretical approach on self-efficacy beliefs to positively influence men with a risk to sexually abuse children. Aggress Violent Behav. 2015;25(A):104–12.

Chapter 14
Non-paraphilic Hypersexual Disorder

Fritjof von Franqué, Verena Klein, and Peer Briken

Introduction

One major theoretical debate in sex research is the conceptualization of high frequent (non-paraphilic) sexual behavior. As a consequence, different attempts have been made to categorize excessive sexual behavior by using different existing psychopathological categories: Carnes [1] introduced the phrase *sexual addiction* as a mood altering pathological phenomenon connected to a sexual process or sexual event. Coleman [2, 3] proposed the term *sexual compulsivity* characterized as temporary regulation of anxiety and distress provoked by intrusion with sexually obsessive behaviors. The expression *sexual impulsivity* was preferred by Barth and Kinder [4] to designate the inability to control strong sexual wishes or reduce the preoccupation with sexual activity. Kafka [5] finally introduced the concept of *paraphilia-related disorder* defined as the increased expression of not socially deviant sexual fantasies, urges, and behaviors [6].

F. von Franqué, Dipl.-Psych., ECPS • V. Klein, Dipl.-Psych.
P. Briken, M.D., F.E.C.S.M. (✉)
Institute for Sex Research and Forensic Psychiatry, University Medical Centre Hamburg-Eppendorf, Martinistr. 52, Hamburg 20255, Germany
e-mail: f.von-franque@uke.de; vklein@uke.de; briken@uke.de

R. Balon (ed.), *Practical Guide to Paraphilia and Paraphilic Disorders*, DOI 10.1007/978-3-319-42650-1_14

Bancroft and Vukadinovic [7] criticized the conceptualization of excessive sexual behavior by using well-known psychopathological categories. The authors argued that different etiological mechanisms for the same kind of excessive sexual behavior might exist. As a consequence, the descriptive expression *out of control sexual behavior* was preferred by these authors until the different etiological mechanisms were clarified. However, Franqué et al. [8] argued that the phrase *out of control* still suggests a control problem and, for this reason, is not descriptive in nature.

As a part of the revision process of the Fifth Edition of the Diagnostic and Statistical Manual of Mental Disorders (DSM-5), Kafka [6] suggested an operational, criterion-based definition for the so-called *hypersexual disorder*. In addition, the attempt was made to avoid linking diagnosis to existing psychopathological frameworks. Although Kafka's proposal was not included in the DSM-5, it seems highly relevant in clinical contexts, since hypersexual disorder might be a risk factor for sexual violence [9] and persons affected report serious impairment in social functioning [10].

In the following chapter, we provide an overview about the diagnostic criteria and the assessment process, followed by a summary of different empirical findings with an emphasis on the treatment for hypersexual disorder. We give a clinical example and recommendations for treatment providers, reflecting our own clinical practice.

Diagnostic Criteria and Assessment Process

The diagnostic criteria for hypersexual disorder suggested by Kafka [6] can be found in Table 14.1.

As a prerequisite for a comprehensive interview, clinicians should have expertise in psychopathology and especially in human sexuality, including knowledge about different pornography genres and sexual services.

It is important to provide an empathic and supportive atmosphere during the interview. Professionals should feel comfortable while speaking about sexual issues; they should know and be able to regulate their own reactions to certain sexual phenomena. Since shame can be strongly associated with hypersexual disorder [8], uncertainties on the part of the clinicians might otherwise reinforce feelings of shame. In addition, the aims and scope of the interview (e.g., assessment or treatment) should be made transparent as well as the limits of confidentiality (e.g., acute risk for violence or suicide). In general, the exploration of the client is the main source of information. However, anamnestic data from third parties, such as sexual partners and other professionals, can be highly valuable. Such data can only be assessed in agreement with the client.

Important aims of the assessment are the current level of functioning including psychopathological symptoms, family and life history, self-image, sexual and relationship history, past mental illness and substance use problems, psychiatric and psychotherapeutic treatment experiences, potential risk signs for sexual violence and/or self-harming behavior as well as the client's future plans. It is important to note that other mental health problems may co-occur with hypersexual disorder. In the literature, high rates of substance abuse problems, mood and anxiety disorders, paraphilias, personality disorders, post-traumatic stress disorder, and organic pathologies are reported [6, 11]. In addition, an assessment of sexual dysfunction problems is recommended [12, 13]. Therefore, clinicians should be aware of any signs for these co-occurring diagnoses. We recommend that ongoing mental health problems like substance abuse, self-harming behavior, and suicidal impulses are dealt with before considering further assessment and treatment for hypersexual disorder. However, there is evidence that substance use may be treated at the same time as hypersexual disorder (see section "Summary of Evidence").

During the sexuological part of information collection, the following areas should be covered:

- Psychosexual development: child sexuality (e.g., genital stimulation, child to child sexual behavior), age of onset of puberty, sexual fantasies, masturbation, intimate relationships, and sexual contacts; content of sexual interests and sexual orientation

- Experiences with sexual and/or violent abuse in childhood, adolescence, or adulthood (as victim or witness)
- Past and present relationship(s): Frequency, duration, relationship and sexual satisfaction, conflicts, sexual activities within the relationship
- Current sexual behavior: Modality and frequency of sexual fantasies, masturbation and sexual contacts within and outside intimate relationships; sexual interests—including paraphilic content—during masturbation and sexual contacts; pornography use, online sexual activity, sexual services, sexual dysfunctions
- Risk signs for sexual violence: Any actual, attempted, or threatened (sexual) harm to a person or persons, criminal prosecutions, paraphilias with non-consenting persons (especially pedophilia and sadism), problems with behavioral control in different life situations, antisocial attitudes

It is highly important that clinicians distinguish between hypersexual disorder and pseudo-hypersexuality. We use the latter term to describe sexual behavior that does not meet the criteria for hypersexual disorder but is accompanied by sexually oppressive thoughts and attitudes like masturbatory guilt or religious prohibitions. In these cases, clients often can benefit from psycho-education on healthy sexuality. If clients have very rigid attitudes, further treatment interventions may be indicated.

In addition, physical examinations are recommended to exclude somatic conditions which can be associated with hypersexual symptoms (like Klüver-Bucy Syndrom; side effect in L-dopa therapy of morbus Parkinson; prefrontal traumatic brain injury). In certain cases, when there are indicators (e.g., abnormal neurological finding, hair-growth, height) of medical conditions associated with hypersexual symptoms, further somatic findings (e.g., chromosome analysis, sex hormones, and neuroimaging) should be used during the diagnostic process.

Summary of Evidence

Depending on research samples, the conceptualization, and measurement of hypersexuality, studies identified different prevalence rates, varying from 3 to 6%. Higher rates had been found in male participants compared to female participants with a ratio ranging from 2:1 to 5:1 [11, 14].

Regarding the treatment of hypersexual disorder, several reviews were published, focusing on theoretical typologies and conceptualizations [15, 16], pharmacological [17–19] and psychotherapeutic interventions [8, 19–21].

Naficy et al. [18] focused on the evaluation of pharmacological effects in treating hypersexual symptoms. In their systematic review, the authors identified seven studies that analyzed the effects of selective serotonin reuptake inhibitors (SSRI), other antidepressants/mood stabilizers, and the opiate antagonist naltrexone. Among these, six studies reported a reduction of hypersexual symptoms. However, according to the authors, very limited conclusions can be drawn from these findings due to conceptional and methodological problems, such as selection biases and especially poor research designs. Interestingly, in the study with the highest research standards [22], pharmacological treatment with SSRI compared to placebo medication was superior in only 3 out of 14 outcome measures. Nevertheless, hypersexual symptoms were significantly reduced in both groups. Naficy et al. [18] did not include the treatment with antiandrogens, although Safarinejad [23] reported effective results with triptorelin (analog of GnRH).

Research on the efficacy of psychotherapeutic interventions is characterized by similar methodological limitations. In their systematic review on pharmacological and psychotherapeutic interventions, Hook et al. [19] identified 14 publications. Among these, eight studies investigated the impact of cognitive behavioral therapy, acceptance and commitment therapy, experiential therapy, motivational interviewing and art therapy on hypersexual disorder. The remaining studies focus on pharmacological effects and are included in the review mentioned above. Most of the psychotherapeutic approaches included in the literature review took place within a group setting. Although Hook et al. [19] reported a reduction in hypersexual symptoms in the majority of studies, the authors suggest that results should be interpreted with caution due to limitations similar to the ones mentioned by Naficy et al. [18]. A more in-depth review of the techniques used is provided by Franqué et al. [8]. Finally, Grubbs et al. [21] focused on new treatment studies since 2012. Only one article was found [24] examining the effects of psychotherapy in a sample of individuals with hypersexual disorder compared to participants with hypersexual and substance abuse disorder. Treatment of both groups consisted of individual therapy, group therapy, 12-step support, recovery planning, and psychosocial education, though group therapy and 12-step support were more intense for the second group. In both treatment arms, significant gains in behavioral regulation, sexual impulse control, and general psychological well-being were reported 6 months after treatment. Grubbs et al. ([21], p. 209) concluded "substance use and hypersexual behavior may be effectively addressed concurrently," while prior research recommended a sequential approach, starting with the treatment of substance use problems. Nevertheless, the same methodological limitations already mentioned (sample selection bias, lack of specific information regarding treatment techniques) apply to this analysis.

Overall the current state of research on treating hypersexual disorder is still limited. Further treatment studies with greater rigor and control are needed, since the field is still in its initial stage.

Clinical Example

Dave was a 30-year-old man, who sought treatment, since he used to spend more than 5 h/day in sex chats, while masturbating once or twice daily. He was engaged in sexual conversations on the internet during the whole day. As a compensation of his time loss, he regularly came home late. Dave became estranged from his wife, who was often already fallen asleep due to her job and taking care of their 3-year-old daughter. She did not know about Dave's sexual activities. According to him, she criticized him very often, since he did not fulfill his family obligations. The couple did not have sex for the duration of almost 3 years. Dave felt ashamed because of the situation and his behavior. In reaction to that, he often started chatting and masturbating until 2 or 3 O'clock in the morning.

Dave was born in a big harbor city. When he was 10 years old, his parents got divorced due to his father's alcohol problem. Dave stayed with his mother, who was described as a very achievement-orientated, but emotionally distant woman. He performed well in school, but he never had many friends. At the age of 11, he hit puberty and started with masturbation, mainly three or four times a week. He imagined that female students from higher levels introduced him to sex. Dave thought himself to be exclusively heterosexual. When Dave was 17 years old, he became the victim of a sexually violent situation during a sport trip. After he had fallen asleep in the boys' dormitory, several unknown persons covered his eyes with a blindfold, fixated and gaged him and pulled down his sleeping pants to slap his genitals. Before they left him, they threatened him not to take off the blindfold. To this day, intrusive thoughts of the incident continue to trigger anxiety in Dave. As a compensation strategy, Dave started masturbating every time memories of the event resurfaced. Since then, the frequency of masturbation increased to six to ten times/week.

After having successfully finished school, Dave began to study. During that time, he started having his first intimate relationship. In total, Dave reports 12 intimate partners in the past. However, he always encountered conflicts in relationships that arose from frequent sexual activities. Female partners often felt pressed, when Dave hoped to have sex more than 7 times/week. His masturbatory rates decreased, as long as female partners were interested in consensual sexuality.

When Dave was 24 years old, he finished his studies with excellence and started to work. At the same age he met his future wife. A year later, they moved together and got married. Dave was very satisfied with their relationship during the first 3 years. The couple had intercourse nearly every day, while Dave masturbated rarely. Then, his wife got pregnant. She refused to go on having sex as frequently as before, but was still interested in sexuality. Since Dave suffered from these changes, the couple had massive disputes. The situation escalated 6 months after the birth of Dave's daughter: His wife demanded couple therapy but Dave refused to participate. Since then, sexuality within the relationship has stopped and Dave started with sexual chats.

Recommendations

As long as best practice guidelines for the treatment for hypersexual disorder are not available, we recommend a prioritization of treatment goals during the assumed phases of (1) stabilization, (2) clarification, (3) coping, and (4) transfer. According to this view, these different periods build on one another. This approach is meant to be flexible. With respect to the individual client, it is possible to start with a later phase or to return temporarily to a completed section. In the following, we will present each phase in more detail.

Stabilization

During the first phase, all interventions are aimed at increasing the capacity for further treatment interventions. Clinicians should manage any acute risk signs for (sexual) violence or self-harming behavior with priority. In these cases, a proper risk assessment is recommended. Sometimes, crisis intervention in a psychiatric hospital may be necessary. Typical interventions in this phase are the implementation of therapeutic commitments in written form, situational control techniques as well as the activation of protective places, persons and activities against sexual acting out. Whenever clients suffer from intrusive thoughts or other forms of traumatic symptoms, we provide stress regulation skills. According to our experience, drug treatment with an SSRI medication can be a great supplement, but should, however, not be used as a stand-alone alternative. Besides, the activation of the client's resources seems to be a very important treatment goal [25]. Lots of clients feel so embarrassed, that they can hardly assess their own strengths. As a consequence, we use parts of a self-esteem training [26]. Finally, the implementation of a good therapeutic alliance provides the basis for any kind of therapy. Clients gain new experiences which may be very helpful in solving their problems (for example, if clients have intimacy deficits). For building such an alliance, empathy is a very solid strategy [27]. According to the therapeutic background (e.g., cognitive behavioral or psychodynamic approaches), other strategies might also be fruitful.

Clarification

In the second phase, a more solid understanding of the problematic behavior should be reached. At the beginning, this can be accomplished through behavioral analysis or other procedures for extracting distal and proximal factors. We encourage clients to do such an analysis, whenever hypersexual symptoms occur in order to learn from each incident. Even more central is the functional analysis of the given behavior. As a framework, we take into consideration different typologies [28, 29], according to which functional causes may be (1) pleasure and sensation seeking, (2) reducing tension and anxiety, (3) avoiding negative emotions, (4) coping with boredom, (5) reducing social distance/isolation, or (6) enhancing social approval. Together with the client, the function of hypersexual behavior should be evaluated. Sometimes, this process requires the client's tolerance of aversive states. Therefore, therapists should alternate clarification techniques with resource activation to avoid resistance and dropouts. At the end of the process, an individual case formulation should be developed. Interventions during the next section should be adapted to this hypothesis. Previously the motivational situation should be taken into account. Usually clients are ambiguous in giving up their hypersexual patterns, since, according to the functional analysis, these patterns have positive short-term consequences. We use the cost benefit analysis [26, 30] or chair techniques [31] to evaluate such ambivalence. Strategies from motivational interviewing [30] may also apply. Whenever the client has decided to change, we move to the next section.

Coping

In the third phase, clients learn central skills tuned to their problems. In the case of some clients, we mainly focus on teaching problem-solving as a strategy of stress management [26]. For other clients, coping with different negative emotions or impulsivity might be the central task. We give psychoeducation about emotions and use mindfulness-based approaches [32] as well as experiential methods [27] to implement improved self-regulation skills. This regularly involves the activation of negative emotions. Sometimes we give therapeutic homework, for example, writing emotional diaries or letters [33]. Some clients struggle with intimate relationship problems. We focus on communicative skills and the improvement of intimacy to heighten relationship satisfaction [34, 35]. When appropriate, sexual education and skills for healthy couple sexuality [36] are provided. For this task, we prefer to work in a couple setting, if both partners are willing to participate. Finally, we help some clients with facing and controlling their fear of (sexually) traumatic experiences. In these cases, we use techniques of narrative exposure therapy [37].

Transfer

In the end, we try to transfer acquired skills into individual contexts [26]. We therefore develop future plans with our clients and encourage them to use their new strategies in order to achieve their personal goals. Particular care shall be taken regarding the management of recurrent hypersexual symptoms and its triggering problems. We provide information that stress could reactivate these behavioral patterns. Clients should be prepared for such situations so that they will not fall into catastrophic thinking but address current issues with the help of their new skills or social support, including therapists. We remind clients to use each new incident as an opportunity to learn something important regarding their self-management. Occasionally, subsequent improvements of the applied strategies are needed. Usually, there is a need for motivational techniques to help clients with a lack of patience. Sometimes participation in community self-help groups is helpful, too.

Conclusion

- Different terms have been used to describe high frequent non-paraphilic sexual behavior. At the moment, this pattern might be best described by Kafka's operational criterion-based definition of hypersexual disorder, since the defining symptoms are not linked to existing psychopathological frameworks.
- For the diagnostic process, clinicians should be able to conduct a comprehensive clinical interview and should feel comfortable with explicitly talking about sexual issues. They should be informed about different forms of sexual interests and behaviors.
- Although in recent years there is a growing body of research focusing on effective approaches to treat hypersexual disorder, our current knowledge is limited due to conceptional and methodological limitations.
- For this reason, there are as of now no best treatment guidelines available. That is why we recommend a flexible approach with a prioritization of treatment goals within various treatment phases. We propose a differentiation of the psychotherapeutic process into the sections (1) stabilization, (2) clarification, (3) coping, and (4) transfer. As a

key task, treatment providers should be able to develop an individual hypothesis regarding the genesis and function of hypersexual disorder and to adapt their interventions to this individual case formulation on the basis of good therapeutic alliance.

Appendix

TABLE 14.1 Proposed diagnostic criteria for hypersexual disorder

A. Over a period of at least 6 months, recurrent and intense sexual fantasies, sexual urges, or sexual behaviors in association with 3 or more of the following 5 criteria
A1. Time consumed by sexual fantasies, urges, or behaviors repetitively interfere with other important (non-sexual) goals, activities, and obligations
A2. Repetitively engaging in sexual fantasies, urges, or behaviors in response to dysphoric mood states (e.g., anxiety, depression, boredom, irritability)
A3. Repetitively engaging in sexual fantasies, urges, or behaviors in response to stressful life events
A4. Repetitive but unsuccessful efforts to control or significantly reduce these sexual fantasies, urges, or behaviors
A5. Repetitively engaging in sexual behaviors while disregarding the risk for physical or emotional harm to self or others
B. There is clinically significant personal distress or impairment in social, occupational, or other important areas of functioning associated with the frequency and intensity of these sexual fantasies, urges, or behaviors
C. These sexual fantasies, urges, or behaviors are not due to the direct physiological effect of an exogenous substance (e.g., a drug of abuse or a medication)

Specify if:
Masturbation, Pornography, Sexual Behavior with Consenting Adults, Cybersex, Telephone Sex, Strip Clubs, Other

References

1. Carnes P. Out of the shadows: understanding sexual addiction. Minneapolis: CompCare; 1983.
2. Coleman E. Sexual compulsivity: definition, etiology, and treatment considerations. J Chemical Depen Treatment. 1987;1:189–204.
3. Coleman E. Is your patient suffering from compulsive sexual behavior? Psychiatric Ann. 1992;22:320–5.
4. Barth RJ, Kinder BN. The mislabeling of sexual impulsivity. J Sex Marital Ther. 1987;13:15–23.
5. Kafka MP. Update on paraphilias and paraphilia-related disorders. Curr Affect Illn. 1993;12:4–8.
6. Kafka MP. Hypersexual disorder: a proposed diagnosis for DSM-V. Arch Sex Behav. 2010;39:377–400.
7. Bancroft J, Vukadinovic Z. Sexual addiction, sexual compulsivity, sexual impulsivity, or what? Toward a theoretical model. J Sex Res. 2004;41(3):225–34.
8. Franqué F v, Klein V, Briken P. Which techniques are used in psychotherapeutic interventions for nonparaphilic hypersexual behavior? Sex Med Rev. 2015;3(1):3–10.
9. Hanson RK, Harris AJR. Where should we intervene? Dynamic predictors of sex offence recidivism. Crim Justice Behav. 2000;21:187–202.
10. Reid RC, Carpenter BN, Hook JN, Garos S, Manning JC, Gilliland R, Cooper EB, McKittrick H, Devtian M, Fong T. Report of findings in a DSM-V field trial for hypersexual disorder. J Sex Med. 2012;9(11):2868–77.
11. Tripodi F, Giuliani M, Petruccelli I, Simonelli C. Hypersexual behavior. In: Kirana PS, Tripodi F, Reisman Y, Porst H, editors. The EFS and ESSM syllabus of clinical sexology. Amsterdam: Medix Publisher; 2013. p. 1144–82.
12. Klein V, Jurin T, Briken P, Stuhlhofer S. Erectile dysfunction, boredom and hypersexuality among coupled men from two European countries. J Sex Med. 2015;12(11):2160–7.
13. Sutton KS, Stratton N, Pytyck J, Kolla NJ, Cantor JM. Patient characteristics by type of hypersexuality referral: a quantitative chart review of 115 consecutive male cases. J Sex Marital Ther. 2014;6:1–18.
14. Briken P, Habermann N, Berner W, Hill A. Diagnosis and treatment of sexual addiction: a survey among German sex therapists. Sex Addict Compulsivity. 2007;14:131–43.

15. Cantor JM, Klein C, Lykins A, Rullo JE, Thaler L, Walling BRA. Treatment-oriented typology of self-identified hypersexual behavior referrals. Arch Sex Behav. 2013;42:883–93.
16. Rosenberg KP, Carnes P, O'Connor S. Evaluation and treatment of sex addiction. J Sex Marital Ther. 2014;40:77–91.
17. Marshall LE, Briken P. Assessment, diagnosis, and management of hypersexual disorders. Curr Opin Psychiatry. 2010;23(6):570–3.
18. Naficy H, Samenow CP, Fong TW. A review of pharmacological treatments for hypersexual disorder. Sex Addict Compulsivity. 2013;20(1–2):139–53.
19. Hook JN, Reid RC, Penberthy JK, Davis DE, Jennings DJ. Methodological review of treatments for nonparaphilic hypersexual behavior. J Sex Marital Ther. 2014;40(4):294–308.
20. Briken P, Hill A, Berner W. Hypersexuality: clinical aspects. In: Aboujaoude E, Koran LM, editors. Impulse control disorders. Cambridge: Cambridge University Press; 2010. p. 197–212.
21. Grubbs JB, Hook JN, Griffin BJ, Davis DE. Evaluating outcome research for hypersexual behavior. Curr Addict Rep. 2015;2:207–13.
22. Wainberg ML, Muench F, Morgenstern J, Hollander E, Irwin TW, Parsons JT, et al. A double-blind study of citalopram versus placebo in the treatment of compulsive sexual behaviors in gay and bisexual men. J Clin Psychiatr. 2006;67:1968–73.
23. Safarinejad MR. Treatment of nonparaphilic hypersexuality in men with a long-acting analog of gonadotropin-releasing hormone. J Sex Med. 2009;6:1151–64.
24. Hartman LI, Ho V, Arbour S, Hambley JM, Lawson P. Sexual addiction and substance addiction: comparing sexual addiction treatment outcomes among clients with and without comorbid substance use disorders. Sex Addict Compulsivity. 2012;19:284–309.
25. Grawe K. Neuropsychotherapy. How the neurosciences inform effective psychotherapy. Mahwah: Lawrence Erlbaum; 2006.
26. Marshall WL, Marshall LE, Serran GA, O'Brien MD. Rehabilitating sexual offenders. A strength based approach. Washington, DC: American Psychological Association; 2011.
27. Elliot R, Watson JC, Goldmann RN, Greenberg LS. Learning emotion-focused therapy: the process-experiential approach to change. Washington, DC: American Psychological Association; 2004.

28. Laws DR, Ward T. Desistance from sex offending. Alternatives from throwing away the keys. New York: Guilford; 2011.
29. Daffern M, Howells K. The function of aggression in personality disordered patients. J Interpers Violence. 2009;24:586–600.
30. Miller WR, Rollnick S. Motivational interviewing. Helping people change. 3rd ed. London: Guilford; 2012.
31. Sachse R, Langens TA, Sachse M. Klienten motivieren. Therapeutische Strategien zur Stärkung der Änderungsbereitschaft. [translated: Motivating clients. Therapeutic strategies for strengthening the willingness to change]. Bonn: Psychiatrie-Verlag; 2012.
32. Kabat-Zinn J. Mindfulness meditation: what it is, what it isn't, and it's role in health care and medicine. In: Haruki Y, Ishii Y, Suzuki M, editors. Comparative and psychological study on meditation. 2nd ed. Netherlands: Eburon Publishers; 2007. p. 161–9.
33. Pennebaker JW. Opening up: the healing power of expressing emotions. New York: Guilford; 2012.
34. Schnarch D. Constructing the sexual crucible: an integration of sexual and marital therapy. New York: Norton; 1991.
35. Sachse R, Breil J, Fasbender J. Klärungsorientierte Paartherapie [translated: Clarification-orientated couple therapy]. Göttingen: Hogrefe; 2013.
36. McCarthy B, McCarthy E. Sexual awareness: your guide to healthy couple sexuality. New York: Routledge/Taylor & Francis; 2012.
37. Schauer M, Neuner F, Elbert T. Narrative exposure therapy. A short-term treatment for traumatic stress disorders. 2nd ed. Cambridge: Hogrefe; 2012.

Chapter 15
Emerging Issues: Compulsive Online Sexual Behaviors

Gabriel Tobia and Waguih William IsHak

Introduction

With the increasing public access to the World Wide Web in the 1990s came the availability of online sex [1] which to this day still represents a sizable portion of internet traffic and income. As a subtype of online sexual activity, "cybersex" is defined as using the internet to engage in sexually gratifying activities [2]. It includes a wide array of behaviors such as viewing erotic or pornographic images; sharing explicit details of one's sex life, including pictures or descriptions of oneself or one's partner; interacting with anonymous partners through forums, chat rooms, or blogs; interacting with sex workers online; meeting potential sexual partners with

G. Tobia, M.D.
Department of Psychiatry and Behavioral Neurosciences, Wayne State University, Tolan Park Medical Building, 3901 Chrysler Service Drive, Suite 5-A, Detroit, MI 48201, USA
e-mail: gtobia@med.wayne.edu

W.W. IsHak, M.D., F.A.P.A. (✉)
Department of Psychiatry and Behavioral Neurosciences, Cedars-Sinai Medical Center, 8730 Alden Drive, Thalians E-132, Los Angeles, CA 90048, USA
e-mail: Waguih.ishak@cshs.org

R. Balon (ed.), *Practical Guide to Paraphilia and Paraphilic Disorders*, DOI 10.1007/978-3-319-42650-1_15

the prospect of an offline relationship; as well as engaging in wanted/unwanted sexually explicit contacts through email, social media, or other online resources [3]. The seemingly unlimited availability of sexual material online, its relative affordability, compounded with the perceived anonymity it provides, has produced what some researchers called a new "sexual revolution" [4]. These characteristics of the internet, in addition to the social values, cultural beliefs, and physical hindrances associated with the world outside the World Wide Web, has contributed to paraphilics and other sexual minorities being "forced online" [5].

Despite the popular media's focus on problematic sexual behavior, it should be noted that the vast majority of online sex users did not suffer significant negative consequences [6]. Although a large number of people engage regularly or sporadically in online sexual activity, the majority do so in moderation [4] and it has been estimated that 83 % of users reported no difficulties in their life related to such activities [6]. Nevertheless, the emergence of online sex may have brought on deleterious consequences to some users, especially those who are likely to be obsessively preoccupied and who persist in online sexual behavior despite negative consequences [7, 8]. Online sexual behaviors become problematic when they lead to negative repercussions legally, medically, financially, occupationally, in relationships, as well as on a personal level [2]. Finally, online sexual compulsivity is defined a "loss of control" over the ability to regulate online sexual activity, leading to negative consequences in the individual's professional, social, and recreational life [2]. Consequences of these problematic behaviors may arise from an isolated incident or a pattern of behavior, and the repercussions may range from feelings of guilt, to a negative impact on relationship and family, or acquiring a sexually transmitted infection [2]. Other potential consequences include criminal pursuit for accessing or sharing illicit pornographic material online most notably child pornography as well as loss of interest in "ordinary" sexual activity with the user's usual partner [9]. Compulsive online sex may also lead to adverse consequences at work, as it is estimated that about 70 % of online sex occurs on weekdays between 9:00 AM and 5:00 PM, which is the workday for many businesses and institutions [7]. Additionally, in the online world as in the offline one, while many paraphilic behaviors are unconventional but harmless, some become destructive, particularly when involving unsuspecting or unwilling participants [5].

Clinical Situation

L.R. is 32-year-old married male who works at an advertising agency as an executive. Since adolescence he has struggled with periods of increasing sexual behaviors such as repeated and prolonged use of pornographic material with excessive masturbation, as well as repeated and prolonged episodes of unprotected sexual encounters with prostitutes and strangers. L.R. sought treatment for his condition and was started on fluoxetine 20 mg daily in addition to attending a 12-step program about 2–3 times per week. L.R. got married 5 years prior to presentation, discontinued his fluoxetine due to sexual side effects, dropped out of his 12-step program, and limited his behavior to online pornography followed by excessive masturbation using his computer, tablet, and smartphone. However, his behavior was escalating to a degree that he would spend hours at work watching pornography on his computer, with frequent visits to the restroom to masturbate. L.R.'s wife noticed that he was disinterested in being physically intimate with her, citing that he was exhausted and was stressed from work. Indeed, his performance at the agency was on the decline, and his viewing of online pornography at work was accidentally discovered. Feeling ashamed of his behavior, he eventually confessed to his wife and asked for her help to seek treatment 2 years ago. The psychiatric evaluation revealed an underlying major depressive disorder and generalized anxiety disorder. Biopsychosocial treatments were then initiated and included mirtazapine, which was increased to 45 mg daily to avoid weight gain and sedation, as well as enrolling in Sexual Compulsives Anonymous. He had to take a brief medical leave from work and was welcomed back as he was gaining more control over his sexual behaviors. Naltrexone 50–100 mg daily was also considered as an alternative medication in case the above regimen with mirtazapine failed since the patient had suffered from anorgasmia while on other SSRIs. In the past year he has been in full remission from sexual behaviors, depression, and anxiety.

Diagnostic Criteria

A single sexual behavior cannot determine whether an individual is compulsive or not, especially as some of the most common of these behaviors, such as masturbation, may not be even problematic for most people [2]. However, sexual behaviors become problematic when three general criteria are present: obsession, compulsion, and consequences of the behavior [10]. The DSM-5 defines obsessions as recurrent and persistent thoughts, urges, or impulses that are experienced, at some time during the disturbance, as intrusive and unwanted, and that in most people cause marked anxiety or distress. The individual attempts to ignore or suppress them or neutralize them by some other thought or action [11]. According to Schneider et al., compulsion occurs when the individual perceives that he has lost "freedom to choose whether to stop or engage in a behavior" [10]. Other considerations include the frequency of the behavior [12] and the desire to reduce or stop said behavior [2]. One proposed diagnostic criterion of compulsive use is spending 11 h or more per week on online sex [6]. The last important factor is the persistence of behavior despite negative consequences [2]. Kafka et al. had proposed the diagnosis of Hypersexual Disorder to be included in the DSM-5 [13]. Although the proposal was eventually rejected, the diagnostic criteria that he suggested remain of interest, especially as compulsive online sexual behaviors would have been classified as a subtype of this condition had it been retained. The diagnostic criteria delineated are, over a period of 6 months, "recurrent and intense sexual fantasies, sexual urges, or sexual behaviors in association" with three or more of the following criteria: "time consumed by sexual fantasies, urges or behaviors repetitively interferes with other important (non-sexual) goals, activities and obligations"; "repetitively engaging in sexual fantasies, urges or behaviors in response to dysphoric mood states"; engaging in these behaviors "in response to stressful life events"; repetitive but unsuccessful efforts to control these behaviors; and finally "repetitively engaging in sexual behaviors while disregarding the risk for physical or emotional harm to self or others." Additionally, there must be "clinically significant personal distress or impairment in social, occupational, or other important areas of functioning," and these behaviors must not be caused by an exogenous substance such as a medication or a drug of abuse. Kafka also included the following specifiers: masturbation, pornography, sexual behavior with consenting adults, telephone sex, strip clubs, as well as the condition at hand, cybersex [13]. In addition to the aforementioned diagnoses, online sexual behaviors may fall under the general category of paraphilic disorders if they fulfill one of two conditions: either the patients "feel personal distress about their interest and not merely distress resulting from society's 'disapproval'," or they "must have a sexual desire or behavior that involves another person's psychological distress, injury, or death, or a desire for sexual behaviors involving unwilling persons or persons unable to give legal consent" [11].

Summary of Evidence

Despite the ubiquity of online sex and extensive media reporting on its negative consequences [14], research on this topic remains scarce and controversial. One study estimates the proportion of problematic users at 17 % [6] while one Swedish study found the number to be less than 10 % [15]. In one study, around 9 % of participants believed that their online sexual behavior was out of control and 10 % felt addicted to both sex and the internet [2]. Of the patients seeking treatment for compulsive online sex, between one-third [2] and one-half were women [16]. A study conducted by Cooper et al. identified three subtypes of online sexual compulsivity: The "Depressive" type uses internet sex as a form of escape from depression. The "Stress-Reactive" type uses internet sex to relieve high levels of stress. The "Fiction and Fantasy" type uses internet sex in order to fulfill sexual desires and as an escape from the daily routine of life [17]. Further studies have attempted to classify pathological online sexual behaviors based on their etiology and linking them to already established sexual disorders, partly as a way to better organize treatment. Some researchers classified compulsive online sexual behavior as a form of sexual addiction [7, 18]. Sex has been likened to a substance of addiction as patients reported withdrawal, tolerance, and spending large amounts of time looking for, engaging in, or recovering from sex. This may also explain why patients with sex addiction respond to 12-step programs [18]. As a form of addiction, compulsive online sex follows four steps: preoccupation, ritualization, compulsive sexual behavior, and unmanageability and despair. Other addictive behaviors such as substance abuse disorders, gambling disorders, or eating disorders may coexist with compulsive online sexual behaviors [3]. Related to the addiction model, the compulsive model proposes that sexual thoughts, images, or impulses can become obsessive for some people to the point of leading to compulsive, repetitive engagement in sexual activity to reduce anxiety [18]. Compulsive sexual behavior could also be described as an impulse control disorder, akin to pyromania. Following this model, the desire for sex can be viewed as an impulse that is extinguished by engaging in excessive repeated sexual activity followed by significant remorse. This model is supported by the high comorbidity of compulsive online sexual behaviors with gambling [3]. Other writers explored gender differences, paraphilias, and loner subtypes as characteristics of compulsive online sex users [19]. Compulsive online sex has been described as maladaptive coping, conditioned behavior, dissociative reenactment of life trauma, and courtship disorder [3]. Maladaptive coping occurs when the individual attempts to use this behavior to cope with overwhelming stress, anxiety, or depression [19]. In fact, depression, dysthymia, and anxiety are very frequent comorbidities in these individuals [20], as described in the above clinical situation. Additionally, it has been posited that both classical and operant conditioning may guide the development of certain sexual preferences as well as the progression of behavior through time, although the issue remains controversial [3, 21–23]. Dissociative reenactment of life trauma may occur with a history of childhood sexual abuse, possibly as a form of conditioning [3]. More importantly, compulsive online sexual behavior has been described as fundamentally a courtship disorder, in which sexual information and decision-making is disrupted, distorted, or misplaced [3]. The evidence for treatment of problematic online sexual behaviors remains scarce and controversial. One study showed that Cognitive Behavioral Group Therapy, including motivational interviewing techniques and psychoeducation, was associated with a decrease of depressive symptoms and increased quality of life in patients with problematic online sexual behaviors, but the behaviors themselves remained unchanged [24]. Other studies using Acceptance and Commitment Therapy [25] and online-based psychoeducation intervention [26] have shown benefit for some patients.

Recommendations for Treatment

Treatment of compulsive online sexual behavior must be tailored depending on the presentation, etiology, and comorbid conditions. When psychopharmacological treatment is necessary, SSRIs such as fluoxetine (60–80 mg per day) or fluvoxamine (100–200 mg per day) are the treatment of choice. Clomipramine (150–300 mg per day) is also effective. Some case reports suggest naltrexone (at 50–100 mg per day) as being effective [18]. When present, comorbid psychiatric illnesses, such as anxiety and mood disorder, as well as substance use disorders, must be treated appropriately, either with antidepressants, psychotherapy, or both. In the context of offender behavior, some internet-based paraphilic disorders such as pedophilia can be addressed pharmacologically, as described elsewhere in this book. Dissociative reenactment as a result of life trauma may be addressed through counter-conditioning [27] as well as other therapy modalities. Relational interventions such as couples and group therapies can be attempted in order to address a courtship disorder and reconstruct distorted or damaged sexual decision-making schemas, as well as reinstating relational boundaries [3]. Finally, relapse prevention may be managed by a combination of cognitive and behavioral interventions, such as behavioral contracts. Psychoeducation is key to breaking the cycle of addiction [7]. Some specialists have advocated attending 12-Step groups dedicated to compulsive online sex users, such as Sex Addicts Anonymous among many others [7].

Conclusion

The widespread availability of sexual material online and its ease of access has led some users to develop problematic online sexual behaviors, characterized by obsession, compulsion, and consequences of the behavior. The etiology of these behaviors are manifold, and may include comorbid anxiety and mood disorders, addiction and impulse control disorder, underlying history of life trauma leading to dissociative reenactment, as well as courtship and intimacy disorders. Treatment of these conditions must be adapted to individual case and should address underlying problems as well as relapse prevention.

References

1. Cooper A. The Internet and sexuality: Into the new millennium. J Sex Educ Ther. 1997;22:5–6.
2. Cooper A, Delmonico DL, Griffin-Shelley E, et al. Online sexual activity: an examination of potentially problematic behaviors. Sex Addict Compulsivity. 2004;11:129–43.

3. Southern S. Treatment of compulsive cybersex behavior. Psychiatr Clin North Am. 2008;4:697–712.
4. Cooper A, Boies S, Maheu M, Greenfield D. Sexuality and the Internet: the next sexual revolution. In: Muscarella F, Szuchman L, editors. The psychological science of sexuality: a research based approach. New York: Wiley; 1999. p. 519–45.
5. Rosenmann A, Safir MP. Forced online: push factors of internet sexuality: a preliminary study of online paraphilic empowerment. J Homosex. 2006;51(3):71–92.
6. Cooper A, Delmonico DL, Burg R. Cybersex users, abusers, and compulsives: new findings and implications. Sex Addict Compulsivity. 2000;7:5–29.
7. Carnes P, Delmonico DL, Griffin E. In the shadows of the net: breaking free of compulsive online sexual behavior. Center City (MN): Hazelden; 2001.
8. Schneider J, Weiss R. Cybersex exposed: simple fantasy or obsession. Center City (MN): Hazelden; 2001.
9. Schneider JP. Effects of cybersex addiction on the family: results of a survey. Sex Addict Compulsivity. 2000;7:31–58.
10. Schneider JP. Sex addiction: controversy within mainstream addiction medicine, diagnosis based on the DSM-III-R and physician case histories. Sex Addict Compulsivity. 1994;1(1): 19–44.
11. American Psychiatric Association. Diagnostic and statistical manual of mental disorders. 5th ed. Arlington: American Psychiatric Publishing; 2013.
12. Kafka M. Psychopharmacologic treatments for nonparaphilic compulsive sexual behaviors. CNS Spectr. 2000;5(1):49–59.
13. Kafka MP. Hypersexual disorder: a proposed diagnosis for DSM-V. Arch Sex Behav. 2010;39:377–400.
14. Cooper A, Putnam DE, Planchon LA, Boies SC. Online sexual compulsivity: getting tangled in the Net. Sex Addict Compulsivity. 2004;11:129–43.
15. Månsson S-A, Daneback K, Tikkanen R, Löfgren-Mårtenson L. Love and sex on the internet. Göteborg: University of Gothenburg; 2003 [in Swedish].
16. Delmonico DL, Griffin EJ, Moriarty J. Cybersex unhooked: a workbook for breaking free from compulsive online sexual behavior. Center City (MN): Hazelden; 2001.
17. Cooper A, Griffin-Shelley E, Delmonico DL, Mathy RM. Online sexual problems: assessment and predictive variables. Sex Addict Compulsivity. 2001;8:267–85.

18. IsHak WW, Boyle A. Sexual desire disorders. In: IsHak WW, editor. The guidebook of sexual medicine. Beverly Hills: A&W Publishing; 2008. p. 97–8.
19. Schwartz MF, Southern S. Compulsive cybersex: the new tea room. In: Cooper A, editor. Cybersex: the dark side of the force: a special issue of the *Journal Sexual Addiction & Compulsivity*. New York: Routledge; 2000. p. 127–44.
20. Kafka MP. Update on paraphilias and paraphilia-related disorders. Curr Affect Illn. 1993;12(6):5–13.
21. Letourneau EJ, O'Donohue W. Classical conditioning of female sexual arousal. Arch Sex Behav. 1997;26:63–78.
22. Plaud JJ, Martini JR. The respondent conditioning of male sexual arousal. Behav Modif. 1999;23:254–68.
23. Pfaus JG, Kippin TE, Centeno S. Conditioning and sexual behavior: a review. Horm Behav. 2001;40:291–321.
24. Orzack MH, Ross CJ. Should virtual sex be treated like other sex addictions? Sex Addict Compulsivity. 2000;7:113–25.
25. Twohig MP, Crosby JM. Acceptance and commitment therapy as a treatment for problematic Internet pornography viewing. Behav Ther. 2000;41:285–95.
26. Hardy SA, Ruchty J, Hull TD, Hyde R. A preliminary study of an online psychoeducational program for hypersexuality. Sex Addict Compulsivity. 2010;17:247–69.
27. Keane TM, Albano AM, Blake DD. Current trends in the treatment of post-traumatic stress symptoms. In: Basoglu M, editor. Torture and its consequences: current treatment approaches. New York: Cambridge University Press; 1992. p. 363–401.

Chapter 16 Ethics and the Therapeutic Relationship in the Care of People Living with Paraphilic Disorders

Christina Tara Khan, Tara C. Collins, and Laura Weiss Roberts

The therapeutic relationship is the foundation of mental health practice and becomes the primary tool through which practitioners help elicit and sustain change in the lives of their patients. The principal goal of this relationship is to nurture a strong alliance that advances a patient's health and overall well-being. Through the therapeutic alliance, practitioners work collaboratively with each patient to formulate a treatment plan that will address the problem or issue that is causing distress or impairment. Along this collaborative path, there may be many challenges, complex decisions, and intrusions upon the clinical care process. Throughout all, the clinician must be attentive to the therapeutic aims of the alliance,

C.T. Khan, M.D., Ph.D. (✉) • L.W. Roberts, M.D., M.A.
Department of Psychiatry and Behavioral Sciences,
Stanford University, Palo Alto, CA, USA

National Center for Posttraumatic Stress Disorder, Dissemination and Training Division, Veterans Affairs Palo Alto Health Care System
e-mail: ckhan@stanford.edu

T.C. Collins, M.D., M.P.H.
Department of Psychiatry, University of California, San Francisco, CA, USA

R. Balon (ed.), *Practical Guide to Paraphilia and Paraphilic Disorders*, DOI 10.1007/978-3-319-42650-1_16

while also remaining attentive to the ethical considerations of respect, beneficence, and fairness [1].

In the context of caring for individuals living with paraphilias and paraphilic disorders, the ethical basis of the therapeutic relationship is paramount because of the societal influences and context that may so greatly affect the health needs of these individuals. Stigma, the potential for exploitation, and legal imperatives affect the therapeutic relationship and may greatly shape the context and aims of clinical care.

Ethical aspects of the care of people living with paraphilias and paraphilic disorders have been largely neglected in the clinical and scholarly literature outside the realm of forensics work with sex offenders. In this chapter, we will outline ethically important issues and considerations in providing care to individuals who derive from vulnerable populations and other special considerations when working with patients with paraphilias and related conditions.

Background and Bioethics Principles

From a human rights perspective, all individuals are free and equal in dignity and rights [2]. A human rights approach to health care asserts that all individuals deserve and have the right to equitable physical and mental health services necessary to preserve health. In aspiring to be a humanistic and just society, attention to ethical principles and standards of care are especially important when working with distinct and marginalized populations, including people living with paraphilias and paraphilic disorders.

Fundamental bioethics principles include, among others, respect for persons, autonomy, beneficence and nonmaleficence, integrity, veracity, and the duty to adhere to the law (Table 16.1). Ethical principles find expression in clinical care practices such as informed consent and confidentiality safeguards. In psychiatric care in particular, attention to informed consent is a crucial aspect of establishing trust in the therapeutic alliance and is a foremost consideration in the provision of care [3]. Informed consent is grounded in the

TABLE 16.1 Ethical principles in the care of people with paraphilic disorders [25–30]

Principles	Illustration
Respect for persons	Individuals are treated as autonomous agents. Persons with diminished autonomy are entitled to protections to assist in making reasoned informed choices
Autonomy	Independence of persons that is free from both controlling interferences by others and from personal limitations that prevent meaningful choice. Informed consent to treatment is grounded in autonomy, whereby individuals act intentionally, with understanding, and without controlling influences
Beneficence and non-maleficence	Complementary principles that persons are treated in an ethical manner through: respect for persons, efforts to secure their well-being, the Hippocratic maxim of "do no harm", and efforts to maximize possible benefits and minimize possible harms
Duty to adhere to the law	Providers should adhere to the requirements of the law, regulations, or other governing authorities
Integrity	Promotion of honesty, truthfulness, and accuracy of one's actions
Veracity	Truth-telling, grounded in respect for persons and autonomy
Fairness	The process of decision making for individuals must be fair and just
Neutrality	Absence of decided views or strong feelings. Not taking sides
Objectivity	Persons are cared for without bias by personal feelings or opinions
Impartiality	Equal treatment of persons, without partiality, bias, or prejudice
Justice	All persons are treated equitably and fairly. Fair distribution of resources, including benefits, risks, and costs

principle of autonomy and refers to an ongoing process that involves sharing information important to the patient, clarifying that the patient has the capacity to make decisions surrounding their health, and ensuring that decisions are authentic and uncoerced [1, 3]. In this context, it is of utmost importance in these cases to present a balanced assessment of risks and benefits and to be mindful of the potential for coercion inherent in competing ethical obligations. Confidentiality is a privilege, linked to the right of privacy, accorded to patients in our society [3, 4]. The aim of this privilege in health care is to protect the personal information that is disclosed, observed, or discovered in the course of a patient's care [3].

For patients who are not voluntarily seeking treatment but rather have been referred or mandated to treatment by a court of law, informed consent and confidentiality practices become more complex to fulfill [5]. When a patient declines treatment for a paraphilic disorder, the clinician's duty to adhere to the law may conflict with the professional aim of respecting patient autonomy. From an ethical perspective, to the extent possible, patients should be informed and engaged in the decision-making processes, even if aspects of their voluntariness have been subordinated to the mandates of the law [5]. Similarly, individuals in mandated treatment may not have the same full privilege of confidentiality, although the clinician working with a patient in this situation does have the responsibility to protect the patient's personal information to the extent permitted by law.

When working with individuals from special populations that are marginalized and have multiple and overlapping sources of vulnerability, certain ethical challenges predictably arise. Patients may feel very uncomfortable sharing their deepest concerns, for fear of being ostracized, reported to authorities, or denied care. Creating a context of trust in which patients have confidence that their feelings and needs will be respected and valued can be very difficult. Patients may feel quite vulnerable in this situation. In individuals with paraphilias and paraphilic disorders, sources of vulnerability may relate to common sociodemographic vulnerabilities such as race, socioeconomic status, or resident status, but may also include less common vulnerabilities associated with stigma, sexuality, and legal consequences. When multiple and overlapping sources of vulnerability exist, there is a need for special attention to ethically important features of the patient's care.

Stigma is a grave concern faced when working in the area of mental disorders in general but even more so when dealing with marginalized populations. People with paraphilias and paraphilic disorders are stigmatized via multiple sources: through engagement in behaviors that are considered atypical and unacceptable; through criminal prosecution and imprisonment; through social isolation; and through loss of support from family, partners, and friends. Attention to stigma may require a more careful approach to building the therapeutic relationship, with awareness of the potential hindrances to developing trust. For example, an individual who is an identified member of a vulnerable population may expect negative judgment and disparate treatment from mental health professionals based on the treatment they have experienced from society at large. Simultaneously, the clinician may have strong countertransference feelings to the individual based on the nature of their known prosecuted behaviors, and this may manifest in ways that perpetuate the effects of societal stigma. Careful attention to the impact of stigma on care-seeking and treatment adherence will be crucial as clinicians establish and maintain a therapeutic alliance.

Sexuality is another area of special consideration when working with patients with paraphilias and paraphilic disorders. Sexuality refers to many things, among them biological sex, gender, gender expression, relational sexual orientation, and erotic sexual orientation [6]. Differences in sexuality thus include many dimensions, including partner or object preference. Persons with paraphilias have sexual attractions and preferences that are different from those that are traditionally accepted by society. These include attraction and preferences for children, animals, objects, or other fantasies that are considered atypical. The DSM-5 has made a distinction between paraphilias and paraphilic disorders, indicating that a paraphilia that rises to the level of a "disorder" is one that causes distress or impairment or one whose satisfaction has engendered harm or risk of harm to oneself or others [7]. While limited research has been done in this area, some have argued that people do not voluntarily choose their sexual attraction and preferences [8] and therefore to discriminate against individuals' preferences based on their biology is unfair. Protection of vulnerable individuals who may be exploited in the context of some paraphilias, as a morality and social justice issue, has nevertheless been the prevailing societal view. It is important to be mindful of the potential conflict between biologically driven sexual preferences and morally informed sexual behaviors in the context of broader society when working with patients with paraphilias.

Caring for the Difficult Patient

When caring for patients from any population, practitioners find themselves feeling challenged by certain patient characteristics or behaviors. Clinicians encounter patients whose thoughts, emotions, and behaviors are uncomfortable, disquieting, or even morally repulsive. A clinician may feel challenged by a verbally combative patient who is argumentative or hostile to a member of the treatment team. Another clinician may feel challenged by a patient who has beliefs that are conflicting with the clinician's own moral underpinnings. In these examples, the clinician may feel that the patient is "difficult." Wise and experienced practitioners come to understand that being "difficult" represents a clinical sign—an indication of an underlying condition that may be addressed therapeutically [9, 10].

Caring for difficult patients is an ethical at-risk situation [11], because it is hard to preserve a sense of authentic engagement, to remain professional and "neutral" or objective in clinical decision-making, and to uphold high quality standards of care when strong negative emotions may be affecting the therapeutic relationship [12]. In the context of care for paraphilic disorders, ethical mistakes may occur when the provider is more focused on uncomfortable feelings toward the patient or when the provider is preoccupied with the idea of harm toward potential victims and, as a result, gives insufficient attention to the patient who is in need of care.

Some common countertransference reactions to "difficult" patients experienced by clinicians are to feel overwhelmed, smothered, threatened, or abnormally angry—or to feel unusually accommodating or forgiving, combined with the desire to "rescue" the patient. These emotional reactions may be a response to something specific the patient says or does, or to projective identification from the patient, often an unconscious process [13]. It is valuable to acknowledge the emotional reactions to a patient that bring about a sense that the patient is "difficult" and to utilize this countertransference to guide clinical decision-making. The task of the clinician is to be able to identify and separate out the mix of contributions from the patient and from the clinician that form any particular countertransference response. In the case of patients with paraphilias and paraphilics disorders, sources of countertransference may include the clinician's own moral and religious feelings and beliefs, particularly in the case of paraphilias the clinician considers especially repugnant. By recognizing the transference and countertransference feelings and behaviors in the treatment relationship, the clinician may identify their own potential hindrances to ethical care and help elucidate the patient's internal object and self-representations that come into play not only in the therapeutic relationship but likely also in the outside world. In this way, a clinician may respond therapeutically and help the patient to identify problematic patterns of behavior.

There are different ways to manage countertransference [13]. One is to tolerate the emotional response to a patient: to observe and sit with the feelings, to contain them, and to understand them. Another is to use the countertransference feelings to inform an interpretive understanding of the patient. Third, one might employ judicious use of self-disclosure to identify for the patient what is happening in the interaction. Together, these three ways of managing countertransference may assist in responding therapeutically and moving the patient closer to the collaborative goal of health and well-being.

Evolving Ethical Duties Across the Continuum of Paraphilic Disorders

Throughout the ages and across the world, cultures have imposed limitations on sexual behavior. While controversial, there are some agreed upon concepts of sexually normative behaviors and of sexually aberrant behaviors [14]. Various factors help determine what is considered normative or non-normative, including the degree of consent, the location of the sexual behavior, the nature of the sexual act, whether any distress or harm may occur, the frequency of the type of sexual practice in society, and the degree of distaste felt by others about the particular sexual behavior [14]. Paraphilic disorders are manifested by fantasies, urges, or actual behaviors. Some paraphilias are expressed while others are not. The threshold for distress and the presence of a formal condition that may benefit from intervention often depends on the severity and urgency of the condition. According to the American Psychiatric Association [7], "most people with atypical sexual interests do not have a mental disorder. To be diagnosed with a paraphilic disorder, DSM-5 requires that people with these interests feel personal distress about their interest, not merely distress resulting from society's disapproval; or have a sexual desire or behavior that involves another person's psychological distress, injury, or death; or have a desire for sexual behaviors involving unwilling persons or persons unable to give legal consent."

There are many different approaches to treating paraphilic disorders. Holistic medicine is the art and science of healing that addresses the whole person—body, mind, and spirit [15]. The practice of holistic medicine integrates conventional and alternative therapies to prevent and treat disease, and to promote optimal health. Holistic medicine focuses on patient education and participation in the healing process [15]. Harm reduction treatment strategies focus on reducing harmful consequences associated with various human behaviors. Critics of harm reduction believe that tolerating risky or illegal behavior sends a message that such behaviors are acceptable [16]. Ethical concerns related to these approaches for individuals with paraphilic disorders involve the tension between treating symptoms that negatively impact the patient and implicitly condoning inappropriate and harmful behavior, and not putting enough emphasis upon the real and actual harm caused to others.

Clinicians may have different responsibilities and ethical duties towards patients across the continuum of paraphilic disorders—in medicine and in society at large, these duties are based in part on the degree of harm and/or exploitation of others. Clinicians may undertake different treatment approaches and a sense of differing ethical duties for those with paraphilic disorders that do not involve another person (e.g., transvestic or fetishistic disorder), or are manifested solely by fantasies or urges. In these cases, a guiding principle for treatment may be based more on the level of distress to the individual than on the level of potential harm to society [17]. Clinicians have more salient ethical imperatives in conditions involving harmful behaviors (e.g., masochistic disorder) or engagement of others who may be vulnerable, particularly if the behavior involves children, or is particularly brutal, humiliating, or violent, such as voyeuristic, exhibitionistic, frotteuristic, sadistic, or pedophilic disorders.

Professionals have obligations that extend beyond those to their patients. Physicians must adhere to the law in protecting the health and well-being of the community and must act with integrity in fulfilling their obligations to society [18]. Clinicians caring for patients with paraphilias and paraphilic disorders may find themselves feeling caught between the duty to provide person-centered, ethically informed care, and the duty to administer treatment that is intended to safeguard the rights of others in society, including potential future victims. In most patient care situations, the obligations of the clinician to the patient, the community, and to society are wholly aligned—and, indeed, in the care of many individuals living with paraphilias that are not exploitative or dangerous, one would expect fairly tight alignment in these obligations. In the care of individuals with some paraphilic disorders,

Paraphilia	Not Expressed	Expressed
Not Exploitative of others	Lowest ethical risk Holistic goals of care predominate Usual ethical safeguards*	Low ethical risk Holistic goals of care predominate Usual ethical safeguards*
Exploitative of others	Moderate ethical risk Holistic and harm reduction goals in tension Heightened ethical safeguards**	Highest ethical risk Harm reduction goals predominate Heightened ethical safeguards**

Fig. 16.1 Ethical safeguard-risk alignment model in the context of paraphilia and paraphilic disorders

however, there may well be misalignment between the patient's wishes, the clinician's obligations in promoting health and assuring safety, and adhering to professional commitments to society. Examples include clinical situations in which harm to others is foreseeable and imminent and when treatment is mandated by the courts but the patient is unwilling to comply.

One of us (LWR) has proposed an ethical safeguard-risk alignment model for the care of individuals living with paraphilias and paraphilic disorders (Fig. 16.1) that relates to a risk-safeguard model [19, 20]. This model helps to support sound clinical ethical decision-making in that it seeks to configure more intensive treatment approaches with increasing risk for harm or for ethical mistakes. For a paraphilic disorder that is not expressed and not exploitative of others, the ethical risk is lowest ethical risk, and the usual ethical safeguards may be employed. Conversely, for a paraphilic disorder that is highly exploitative of others, and is also expressed, particularly if to a high degree, the ethical risk involved is the highest, and heightened ethical safeguards and harm reduction goals predominate. In essence, the higher the risk, the higher the safeguards need to be.

In working with vulnerable populations and in working in situations in which there is heightened risk, or both, it is important to engage in series of steps that help improve the rigor of ethical decision-making. Learning to recognize ethical issues, seeking to clarify ethical tensions, gathering additional data or expertise, obtaining supervision or consultation, and safeguarding against errors in judgment are key skills in working in difficult patient care situations (Table 16.2).

Table 16.2 Ethics skills in the care of people with paraphilic disorders

Skills	**Potential applications**
Establish trust and therapeutic rapport	Helps individuals to be more forthcoming with current and past symptoms, which in turn helps professionals to provide more accurate diagnosis and treatment recommendations
Use clear and concise communication with patients, particularly taking into account level of education and culture	Allows for individuals to exercise autonomy and truly participate in the informed consent process
Gather collateral information	Allows for a more thorough assessment, improved accuracy in diagnosis, and more person-centered treatment recommendations. Promotes objectivity, impartiality, beneficence and non-maleficence, among other ethical principles
Identify and manage countertransference	Helps to promote fairness and objectivity
Actively identify potential biases and prejudices	Helps providers to act with objectivity and impartiality
Seek consultation and/or supervision	Helps with managing countertransference. Promotes fairness, neutrality and objectivity. For providers without expertise in paraphilias, helps with the provision of quality care. Helps safeguard against errors in judgment amidst complex ethical decision-making
Consider the values of all stakeholders involved	Promotes justice and respect for persons

(continued)

TABLE 16.2 (continued)

Skills	Potential applications
Strengthen communication, address conflict, and promote problem-solving among members of team	Helps to reduce team conflict, which can greatly impact patient care in a variety of ways, including challenges to ethically sound provision of care
Identify available resources	Promotes fairness and justice in the allocation of limited resources
Develop an understanding of human rights and basic biomedical ethical principles	Helps providers to recognize and address ethical concerns in the care of vulnerable populations
Develop a clear understanding of statutes and mandatory reporting requirements	Facilitates the principle of duty to adhere to the law. Promotes understanding of what is reportable, and what is not. Helps safeguard against errors in judgment amidst complex ethical decision-making
Learn and understand pharmacological and non-pharmacological treatment options, and the evidence supporting them	Provides individuals with an appropriate treatment plan, based on the best available evidence. Supports informed consent and autonomy

Case Discussion

Case 1: Exploitative Paraphilia

Mr. H is a 45-year-old recently divorced, employed man with two adult step-daughters and one teenage son, and no previous psychiatric history, who was involuntarily admitted to an inpatient psychiatric unit after a suicide attempt. Mr. H was the subject of a 3-month investigation by the local Sheriff's Office Crime Scene Investigation and Domestic Violence Sexual Assault Units for suspicion of possessing child pornography. Mr. H's apartment was searched and his computer seized by investigators approximately 1 week prior to his suicide attempt.

Mr. H reported that due to overwhelming anxiety and depression related to his likely future charges and imprisonment, as well as the expected negative response from his family, friends, and coworkers, he had decided to kill himself. Mr. H went to the coast, with a plan to jump off the cliffs in order to end his life. While he was standing on the precipice, the wind picked up, and Mr. H slipped over the edge of the cliff and slid to the rocks below. He suffered some lacerations, abrasions, and contusions, but was not significantly injured and did not lose consciousness. Mr. H slowly made his way up the cliff, and returned to his car, still feeling suicidal. He noticed a picture of his children in his car, and changed his mind and went home. Mr. H called his brother and told him what happened, and Mr. H's brother called 911, the emergency dispatch telephone number in the United States and Canada that may trigger an emergency response.

Initially, during multiple interviews over several days with the inpatient psychiatrist, social workers, and nurses, Mr. H steadfastly maintained that while he did in fact possess and look at child pornography, that was the extent of his behavior. He adamantly denied ever having any physical or electronic contact with children, and denied behaviors such as masturbation and fantasies. Mr. H discussed his own history of physical and sexual abuse perpetrated by his father, including rape, which was confirmed by Mr. H's brother.

Later, after several days in the hospital, Mr. H admitted that he had lied about his suicide attempt. He reported that he was never suicidal, and that he faked an aborted suicide attempt in order to gain support and sympathy from his family. Mr. H went on to report a long history of being sexually attracted to children, both male and female, from about 5 years of age and up. He was also sexually attracted to adults. Mr. H admitted that he had lied about his behaviors surrounding his sexual attraction to children. He eventually discussed masturbating to sexual fantasies about children, and also at times fantasized that he was a child being abused.

Mr. H noted that his child pornography viewing habits had worsened after his divorce, as he was more alone and isolated and "had fewer checks on my habit." Mr. H continued to adamantly deny any electronic or physical contact with children.

A few days prior to discharge, Mr. H again admitted that he had been lying about the extent of his pedophilic activities, and that he had touched his two step-daughters in their vaginal area when they were younger, less than 11 years old, over a decade ago. He reported that this occurred a maximum of six or seven times, while the girls were sleeping, and he does not believe that they were aware of what happened. He also stated that when he was 19 years old, he touched a young girl inappropriately at camp while he was a camp counselor. He denied any other history of touching or engaging in any sexual activity with other children.

Mr. H's admission and treatment raise a host of ethical issues. At the time of his hospitalization, many on Mr. H's treatment team sympathized with him initially, particularly given his history of physical and sexual abuse, and were quite motivated to help improve Mr. H's symptoms of depression and anxiety. However, as the patient began to divulge more and more information that he had previously lied about or withheld, it became increasingly difficult for his providers to maintain neutrality, objectivity, and impartiality, and to abide by the principles of beneficence and non-maleficence. Over time, Mr. H was quite often cast by staff as a "psychopathic, manipulative liar" who could not be trusted and was likely being dishonest about all of his psychiatric symptoms. While most members of his treatment team were able to maintain a professional and courteous demeanor with Mr. H, there were some providers who were not able to do so. The reactions of the professionals to Mr. H led to increasingly difficult interactions amongst the members of the health care team regarding the patient's treatment and length of stay.

The patient's pattern of divulging more and more background information, and contradicting early versions, also led to questions about what to disclose to Mr. H's family and what to report to local authorities. The professionals on the team took very seriously their duty to treat Mr. H, as well as the duty to fulfill mandated reporting requirements related to child sexual abuse, yet there was no evidence that Mr. H was currently harming any children. There was extensive discussion about what to document: what was necessary to include in the medical record, what was pertinent to Mr. H's diagnosis and treatment, and what was superfluous and could cause him harm related to his pending legal troubles. The treatment team faced questions about what their responsibilities were to the patient and what their responsibilities as physicians and other providers were to society, to keep the greater public safe. Many individuals with pedophilic disorder involved in the legal system do not fully disclose their crimes right away. Some questions that arose were if there were more victims or if Mr. H had engaged in more aggravated forms of child sexual abuse that he had not yet disclosed. The team wondered, is it solely up to investigators of the law to attempt to uncover more information during the investigation, or should mental health providers indirectly assist in the investigation with the hope and goal of protecting children?

Mr. H's choice of treatment, particularly pharmacotherapy, also raised several ethical concerns. Initially, to target Mr. H's pedophilic disorder, anxiety, and depression, a decision was made to start fluoxetine, a selective serotonin reuptake inhibitor (SSRI). Case reports and open-label trials have found that SSRIs can be helpful in paraphilic disorders, however there are no existing robust, randomized controlled trials supporting their efficacy [17, 21, 22]. This was discussed in great detail with Mr. H, and he expressed a desire to start fluoxetine. As Mr. H began to disclose additional information, the question of simultaneous hormonal therapy, or chemical castration, arose. Given the time elapsed since his last self-reported violation, it was not clear that chemical castration, with its myriad of side effects and potential adverse events, and its lack of strong evidence as an intervention, was justified [23]. Furthermore in question was whether the initiation of expensive medications requiring monitoring was justified if unlikely to be continued in jail and/or prison, particularly if Mr. H was not enthusiastic about such treatment and may no longer have access to children. Among others, these ethical concerns highlighted the complexity of working with individuals with paraphilic disorders who are exploitative of others.

Case 2: Non-exploitative Paraphilia

Mr. Y is a 32-year-old single, employed man who presented for voluntary outpatient treatment for transvestic disorder. Mr. Y was entering into a new relationship, and was extremely distressed about his strong sexual fantasies and urges to dress in women's lingerie and makeup and, masturbate.

Mr. Y reported several of his past relationships had ended when his significant other discovered his transvestic symptoms. Over the years he had developed overwhelming anxiety, shame, and dread related to his thoughts and behavior, while he simultaneously felt compelled to continue to cross-dress and experienced sexual gratification from this behavior.

Mr. Y had researched paraphilic disorders and treatment online and was very interested in pharmacotherapy, specifically anti-androgen medications. Because Mr. Y's symptoms were not harmful to others and did not lead to criminal activity, psychotherapy (behavioral therapy and/or cognitive behavioral therapy) was recommended, with the possible addition of an SSRI [21]. While there is some evidence to suggest that transvestic disorder may respond best to a 3-pronged approach (therapy, antidepressants, and anti-androgens), as with most paraphilic disorders, the evidence is not strong [24]. Anti-androgens can have significant side effects, including metabolic changes, fatigue, gastrointestinal problems, cardiovascular problems, bone loss, and headaches [23]. Also, there is the risk that the resultant decrease in sexual drive may lead to problems with intimacy in relationships, which Mr. Y was seeking.

In addition to these clinical concerns, Mr. Y had no commercial insurance and had few financial resources for his treatment.

In this case, the ethical issues pertain primarily to defining and fulfilling therapeutic goals, especially in a context of stigma and limited resources. Mr. Y felt his fantasies and urges were so compelling and overwhelming as to significantly lessen his quality of life, however there was no guarantee the recommended treatment would be effective. In recommending appropriate treatment, finding a balance among autonomy, beneficence, and non-maleficence all came into play. Social justice issues were also salient in that access to care was a barrier. Ideally, the care of individuals with non-exploitative paraphilic disorders like Mr. Y will take place in the context of a long-term therapeutic relationship in which difficult issues may be addressed over time and in support of the individual's overall well-being. Such a long-term relationship is not possible in the absence of adequate resources.

Conclusion

Attention to the ethical basis of the therapeutic relationship is central to ethically sound care for people living with paraphilias and paraphilic disorders. These individuals are often marginalized and face many challenges in our society. Though many may view these patients as "difficult," this observation may be better understood as a clinical sign that may be amenable to therapeutic intervention. Paraphilias and paraphilic disorders are different in their nature and impact, and therefore differ in the range of responses that they require, ethically, from clinicians. An ethical safeguard-risk alignment model has been proposed in which more intensive treatment approaches are required in situations of increased potential for harm and ethical mistakes. Strong ethics skills, such as gathering additional information and expertise and seeking consultation, are advisable in caring for vulnerable populations, including individuals living with paraphilias and paraphilic disorders—people who, along with all others, deserve freedom and equality in dignity and rights.

References

1. American Psychiatric Association. APA commentary on ethics in practice. 2015. http://www.psychiatry.org/psychiatrists/practice/ethics. Accessed 17 Mar 2016.
2. United Nations. Universal declaration of human rights. 1952. http://www.bl.uk/collection-items/universal-declaration-of-human-rights. Accessed 17 Mar 2016.
3. Roberts LW, Geppert CM, Bailey R. Ethics in psychiatric practice: essential ethics skills, informed consent, the therapeutic relationship, and confidentiality. J Psychiatr Pract. 2002; 8(5):290–305.
4. Roberts L, Dyer A. Concise guide to ethics in mental health care. Washington, DC: American Psychiatric Publishing; 2004.
5. Mela M, Ahmed AG. Ethics and the treatment of sexual offenders. Psychiatr Clin North Am. 2014;37(2):239–50.
6. Tolman D, Diamond L, editors. APA handbook of sexuality and psychology. Washington, DC: American Psychological Association; 2014.
7. American Psychiatric Association. Diagnostic and statistical manual of mental disorders. 5th ed. Washington, DC: American Psychiatric Publishing; 2013.
8. Berlin FS. Issues in the exploration of biological factors contributing to the etiology of the "sex offender", plus some ethical considerations. Ann N Y Acad Sci. 1988;528:183–92.
9. Roberts LW. Difficult patients. In: Roberts LW, editor. A clinical guide to psychiatric ethics. Arlington: American Psychiatric Publishing; 2016.
10. McCarty T, Roberts LW. The difficult patient. In: Rubin RH, Voss C, Derksen DJ, et al., editors. Medicine: a primary care approach. Philadephia: WB Saunders; 1996.
11. Roberts LW. Ethical use of influence and role of physician in high-risk situations. In: Roberts LW, editor. A clinical guide to psychiatric ethics. Arlington: American Psychiatric Publishing; 2016.
12. Lally MC, Freeman SA. The struggle to maintain neutrality in the treatment of patient with pedophilia. Ethics Behav. 2005; 15(2):182–90.
13. Gabbard GO. Long-term psychodynamic psychotherapy: a basic text. 2nd ed. Washington, DC: American Psychiatric Publishing; 2010.

14. Thibaut F, De La Barra F, Gordon H, Cosyns P, Bradford JMW. The World Federation of Societies of Biological Psychiatry (WFSBP) guidelines for the biological treatment of paraphilias. World J Biol Psychiatry. 2010;11(4):604–55.
15. Trivieri LJ, The American Holistic Medical Association. The American Holistic Medical Association guide to holistic health: healing therapies for optimal wellness. New York: Wiley; 2001.
16. Collins S, Clifasefi S, Logan D, Samples L, Somers J, Marlatt G. Current status, historical highlights, and basic principles of harm reduction. In: Marlatt G et al., editors. Harm reduction: pragmatic strategies for managing high-risk behaviors. New York: Guilford; 2012.
17. Balon R. Controversies in the diagnosis and treatment of paraphilias. J Sex Marital Ther. 2012;39(1):7–20.
18. Williams JR. Medical ethics manual. 3rd ed. Ferney-Voltaire: World Medical Association, Inc.; 2015.
19. Roberts LW. Advancing science in the service of humanity: professionalism and ethical safeguards. JAMA Inten Med. 2015;175(9):1506–8.
20. Roberts LW, Ohayon MM, Kim JP. Ethical issues in biomedical research and clinical training. In: Roberts LW, Reicherter D, editors. Professionalism and ethics in medicine: a study guide for physicians and physicians-in-training. New York: Springer; 2015.
21. Briken P, Kafka MP. Pharmacological treatments for paraphilic patients and sexual offenders. Curr Opin Psychiatry. 2007;20(6):609–13.
22. Lösel F, Schmucker M. The effectiveness of treatment for sexual offenders: a comprehensive meta-analysis. J Exp Criminol. 2005;1(1):117–46.
23. Giltay EJ, Gooren LJG. Potential side effects of androgen deprivation treatment in sex offenders. J Am Acad Psychiatry Law. 2009;37(1):53–8.
24. Gijs L, Gooren L. Hormonal and psychopharmacological interventions in the treatment of paraphilias: an update. J Sex Res. 1996;33(4):273–90.
25. National Commission for the Protection of Human Subjects of Biomedical and Behavioral Research. The Belmont report: ethical principles and guidelines for the protection of human subjects of research. Washington, DC: US Government Printing Office; 1979.
26. Zaidi SH. Ethics in medicine. Cham: Springer International Publishing; 2014.

27. American Medical Association. AMA's code of medical ethics. 2016. http://www.ama-assn.org/ama/pub/physician-resources/medical-ethics/code-medical-ethics.page?ma_guidelines. Accessed 17 Mar 2016.
28. Snyder L. American college of physicians ethics manual, 6th edition. Ann Intern Med. 2012;156:73–104.
29. Beauchamp TL, Childress JF. Principles of biomedical ethics. 7th ed. New York: Oxford University Press; 2013.
30. Halpern J. From detached concern to empathy: humanizing medical practice. New York: Oxford University Press; 2001.

Chapter 17
Legal Issues Involved in the Management of Paraphilic Disorders

Brad D. Booth

Introduction

Many of the named paraphilic disorders inherently bring an increased risk of legal overlap. This includes for individuals suffering from paraphilic disorders, who may face legal prosecution for the behaviors stemming from paraphilic drives. For clinicians, legal issues abound working with individuals with paraphilic disorders. This includes assessing individuals for legal proceedings who have committed sexual offences—sentencing issues, risk assessments, sexually violent predator evaluations, and court mandated treatment. Further, clinicians often act as expert witnesses to advise and educate the courts. Issues can also include the boundaries between the courts and ethics of clinical practice such as forced treatment, involuntary commitment, and facing pressures from the legal process to label individuals "sick" given their actions.

B.D. Booth, M.D., F.R.C.P.C. (✉)
Integrated Forensic Program, Division of Forensic Psychiatry, Department of Psychiatry, Royal Ottawa Mental Health Centre, University of Ottawa, 2nd Floor—Forensics, 1145 Carling Avenue, Ottawa, ON, Canada, K1Z 7K4
e-mail: brad.booth@theroyal.ca

R. Balon (ed.), *Practical Guide to Paraphilia and Paraphilic Disorders*, DOI 10.1007/978-3-319-42650-1_17

While beyond the scope of this volume, there are endless legal, ethical, and historical debates discussing sexual "deviance." Inherent in these controversies are the ethical issues of:

- Autonomy—the right of the person to decide their destiny (e.g., in this case, to do whatever sexually interests them)
- Utilitarian issues—that which serves the greater good (e.g., to prevent moral decline)
- Police power—the right of the State to protect its citizens (e.g., to protect individuals from being either direct or indirect victims of sexual activities of others)
- Natural justice—those that do harm to others should be punished (e.g., a sexual assault on a child causes the child harm and the perpetrator should lose freedom)
- Beneficence and non-maleficence—medical practitioners duty to help patients and do no harm (e.g., to diagnose and treat medical conditions)
- *Parens patriae*—the State's obligation to protect vulnerable individuals (e.g., to protect those who may not know better than to act on their harmful sexual interests)

Societal pressures, including religion and politics, heavily influence the legal and legislative application of these ethical principles. Further complexity arrives from ambiguity around what constitutes "mental illness" and the role of health care providers in helping individuals who are either victims of sexually "inappropriate" behaviors or the perpetrators. The result has been significant disagreement and wide swings in policy around sexual behavior, including within the field of mental health.

Part of the disparity results from blurring and confusion on terminology from citizens, journalists, and law-makers. Individuals working in medicine, mental health, and even in those working regularly with sexual offenders similarly blur definitions. Within this chapter, the following terms are used:

- Sexual act—doing an actual sexual activity, regardless of motivation
- Paraphilic interest—one of many potential drives to do a particular sexual act, defined in the DSM-5; usually considered a "deviant" interest

- Paraphilic disorder—as per DSM-5 are those paraphilic interests which cause distress/dysfunction or rise to actions which interfere with the significant rights of others
- Deviant interest—dysfunctional sexual interest; definitions inherently heavily influenced by societal pressures (e.g., religion, majority opinion, and political influences)
- Illegal sexual act—legislated prohibition against particular sexual activities
- Non-paraphilic sexual disorder—as per DSM-5, realizing sexual disorders may influence sexual behavior (e.g., hypersexuality)

With these definitions, specific sexual acts are defined by legislators as illegal—these laws are influenced by religion and majority interests balanced against other competing ethical principles, particularly autonomy. Thus, in a more conservative societal context, legislators may define many sexual acts as criminal—this could include fellatio, sexual intercourse with someone other than one's spouse, viewing pornography, and participating in homosexual sex. Under a similar structure, forced or violent sex with one's spouse may be deemed as legal, wherein a spouse has universally consented as part of the marital contract or wherein one spouse is the "property" of the other.

In more liberal and advanced societies, there is increased focus on autonomy rights, making many of the aforementioned activities legal. In keeping with autonomy rights, those acts that interfere with an individual's right to their body integrity, sexual acts on non-consenting individuals (including one's spouse), are generally illegal. This can include those acts likely to cause direct physical or psychological harm to the victim.

Regardless of the legal framework, sexual behaviors and paraphilic disorders can have profound legal implications. Forensic mental health workers will often be called to bring a psychiatric perspective to this legal arena for the courts. This includes education about normative sexual activity in addition to the clarification of motivations of offending, risk assessment, and risk management/treatment of these individuals. This chapter will review further the diagnostic issues around paraphilic disorders within a legal context. In addition, the current legal context will be discussed with clinical cases and recommendations.

Diagnostic Criteria

Diagnostic criteria for the paraphilic disorders in the DSM-5 are not without contention. With the development of the DSM-5, further effort has been made to differentiate a paraphilic interest from a disorder (i.e., mental illness).

With the DSM-5, some authors discouraged adding new diagnoses such as pedo-hebephilic disorder, hebephilic disorder, coercive paraphilic disorder, and hypersexual disorder [1–5]. Concerns cited include citing the potential for abuse by the legal system, declaring individuals mentally ill where no illness exists, labelling normative arousal as illness, stigma, and a lack of consensus in the field. Historically, similar concerns have been noted, citing the risk of relying heavily on culture and religion to define disease [6, 7]. Ultimately, the DSM-5 paraphilic disorder criteria have seen relatively few changes from the DSM-IV-TR. One useful change has been to provide further differentiation from paraphilic behaviors and differentiating this from paraphilic disorders.

Paraphilic Disorder Diagnostic Criteria in the Legal Realm

The DSM-5 includes a number of named paraphilic disorders which have been included given the prevalence in clinical situations, whether through medico-legal referrals or through self-referrals. Some bring foreseeable risks for legal problems. The courts often need to gain an understanding of the history of paraphilic diagnoses, the controversies in the area, the diagnostic criteria, and any relative risks conveyed by the diagnoses. Clinicians must ensure they are familiar with this information and should only act as an expert if experienced, trained, and bringing evidence-based practice to the court.

While all paraphilic disorders by definition may cause distress or dysfunction for the individual with the paraphilia, usually legal regulation focusses more on protecting the significant rights of others. Thus, it is useful to subdivide paraphilic disorders by the potential for risk to others. Those with higher risk of profound physical and psychological harm include:

- Pedophilic disorder
- Sexual sadism disorder

In pedophilic disorder, individuals are significantly aroused by pre-pubescent children. Child molesters with pedophilic disorder have an increased risk of recidivism [8]. That said, some authors have questioned the reliability and utility of the pedophilia diagnosis [9–12]. Further, many inexperienced evaluators will equate sexual offending against children with a diagnosis of pedophilia. Alternatively, age of consent will be used to determine pedophilia diagnoses as opposed to arousal to pre-pubescent children. This diagnosis can be interpreted in a stigmatizing manner by the court. Making such a diagnosis prior to a finding of guilt could also unduly influence and bias the court's decisions. The courts and some clinicians do not recognize that these and other psychiatric diagnoses and criteria were established for clinical and research applications by trained clinicians, and not specifically for the needs of the court.

Similar problems come in diagnosing sexual sadism disorder. In this disorder, individuals are aroused to the suffering of non-consenting partners. While rarely this diagnosis occurs in those committing sexual assaults, the courts and evaluators often mistakenly equate sexual assault with sadism. In fact, many individuals committing rape have no abnormal arousal on testing; similarly, arousal to coercive and sadistic themes on phallometric testing can be seen in high numbers of "normal" non-offending individuals [13–15]. An inaccurate label of sexual sadism can also profoundly affect high-stakes evaluations for the court [16]. While important not to mistakenly give this label, the presence of sexual sadism disorder could indicate an increased propensity for severe violence in some offenders [17–19]. Ultimately, evaluators have an ethical and legal responsibility to ensure their skills and knowledge are sufficient to give such opinions to the court.

Outside of pedophilic disorder and sexual sadism disorder, other paraphilic disorders are generally considered less likely to cause profound harm in most victims and instead may lead to nuisance offences. These disorders include:

- Frotteuristic disorder
- Voyeuristic disorder
- Exhibitionistic disorder
- Fetishistic disorder

Frotteuristic disorder may be present in a minority of sexual offenders who are specifically aroused in a paraphilic manner by groping non-consenting strangers. However, this label is often inaccurately given to anyone with a groping offence. Often more likely causes should be considered such as intellectual deficits, impulse control problems, and other sexual issues.

Voyeuristic disorder and exhibitionist disorder are differentiated from their associated behaviors based on intensity and frequency. This is important as some community studies have suggested such behaviors are relatively common in the population [20]. Individuals who are convicted of these offences often have high numbers of previous victims and are at a relatively high risk of recidivism. A minority may progress to more serious offending. Even if they do not, such offences can be quite distressing for victims [21].

Fetishistic disorder in which individuals are highly aroused to nonhuman objects (e.g., leather, lace, fur, shoes, underwear) generally does not lead to direct harm to others. However, driven by paraphilic interests, some authors estimate about 25 % of fetishists will steal their fetish objects (e.g., stealing underwear from victims) [22]. Alternatively, the perpetrator could also have other comorbid more harmful paraphilias. Having one's belongings stolen could cause significant distress to victims, particularly if the culprit breaks into the residence of the victim.

The remaining named paraphilias are unlikely to cause profound harm directly to victims, though bring a potential to indirectly "offend the morality" of society thus causing psychological distress:

- Sexual masochism disorder
- Transvestic fetishism

In the legal arena, clinicians should assist in de-stigmatizing these disorders if the courts incorrectly equate deviancy with risk. If evidenced from the assessment, it may be occasionally useful to highlight the risk for "crossing over" [23] in any of the paraphilic disorders. This phenomenon does not occur universally though could be relevant in some offenders. For example, while the majority of individuals with transvestic fetishism pose no risk, a small number of those committing sexually motivated homicide have comorbid transvestic fetishism [24]. Similarly, a portion of sexual masochists will have comorbid sexual sadism.

The final disorder, "Other specificed paraphilic disorder" could have varying risk of harm for victims in the above categorization. This might include benign interests such as klismaphilia (arousal to enemas) or highly dangerous interests such as biastophilia (arousal to rape) or Erotophonophilia (arousal to murder). Presumably those with paraphilic drives will be at somewhat increased of that offending behavior.

Paraphilic Disorder Criteria Importance and Relationship to Offending

Individuals perpetrating prohibited sexual acts may be influenced by a paraphilic disorder. That said, many individuals perpetrating such acts could have other motivations and influences. For example, bestiality (persons having sexual contact with animals) is still considered illegal in much of North America [25] though some cultures do not prohibit this activity [26]. Regardless of the legality, sexual contact with animals could be motivated by a specific paraphilic disorder,

"Other Specified paraphilic disorder (zoophilia)." This is generally considered to be a sexual disorder in which individuals have recurrent, intense, and often preferential or obligatory arousal to animals. Though this may motivate some individuals committing the offence of bestiality, other possible motivators include intellectual disability, disinhibition by mental illness (e.g., psychosis, mania, brain injury), disinhibition by intoxication, social isolation, lack of a consensual partner, or high sexual drive [27, 28]. At the same time, some individuals with zoophilia may not act on this interest to commit an illegal act. Expert knowledge of the diagnostic criteria and related literature is important and experts should be prepared to challenge misperceptions of the cause of offending and the risk posed by the presence of a particular paraphilia.

In other offending situations, there could be non-paraphilic, frequent or "normal" sexual interests which contribute to offending. For example, sexual arousal to pubescent girls is frequent in non-offending populations [1] and argued to be "normal." Historically the age of consent in some societies has been closely linked to child-bearing ability and not full intellectual maturity. If a jurisdiction sets the age of consent for sexual relationships at 16 years old, as is in the situation in Canada currently, then there is a temptation by the courts and some clinicians to incorrectly give a label of pedophilia to anyone offending against 15-year-old girls despite this being driven by normal biological arousal. The flaw of this is highlighted further when jurisdictions change the age of consent (e.g., to 14 years old, as it was previously in Canada). These individuals would no longer be labelled "ill," despite identical behavior. Some courts have similarly labelled 17-year-old boys who have consensual intercourse with 15-year-old girls as pedophilic despite this again being driven by normal biological arousal. This highlights the tension seen at times between the courts, society, and the medical field; the clinician's role would be to educate the legal system about normative sexuality and avoid becoming a pawn to the court and societal pressures to pathologize individuals.

In a similar vein, some societies have designated homosexual acts as illegal with severe punishment up to and including death. In North American history, this also was the case. In so doing, normal homosexual arousal could be inappropriately pathologized. Indeed, in the past, homosexuality was listed in the Diagnostic and Statistical Manual as an illness. This highlights the need to vigilant about the societal pressure to turn behavior into illness. Canada and most states have not only decriminalized homosexual activity, but also afforded significant protective rights to this population.

Summary of Evidence

Despite the controversies, mental health care and correctional personnel are often in the position of managing the risk of individuals with illegal sexual behaviors—which may or may not be due to a paraphilic disorder; further, many individuals with paraphilic disorders will not offend. Risk management of sexual offenders usually involves some curtailing of liberty interests and autonomy of the offender. The role of health care providers is variable, but should be limited to educating the courts about risk, diagnosis, and treatments and then providing the treatments for mental health issues.

Once the risk of sexual violence has been evaluated, the next step is to evaluate how to manage that risk for that particular offender. Management strategies should be tailored to the offender's risk, needs, and the availability of resources. While there may be societal pressure for harsh sentencing as the only risk management strategy, this narrow approach is financially prohibitive and can put a disproportionate amount of public resources towards unnecessary or ineffective interventions [29].

Management strategies of offenders include:

- External control
- Psychotherapy-based treatments
- Pharmacotherapy treatments
- Treatment of comorbidities

External Control

External control mechanisms are those interventions that generally are imposed by the criminal justice system. Legal strategies include:

- Criminalization of specific behaviors (e.g., illegal to have sexual contact with animals)
- Increased sentence length
- Civil commitment/indefinite sentencing
- Post-release conditions

Criminalization of Specific Behaviors

While this approach may arguably have merit from a legal perspective, clinicians should be careful to separate this from their clinical duties. Clinicians may play a role in educating the courts about paraphilic disorders, offending and risk management strategies. However, clinicians need to be wary of allowing societal and legal pressures from dictating diagnosis and treatment issues. Just because a person embarks on criminal behavior, it does not mean the person is definitely mentally ill or warrants psychiatric intervention. That being said, some individuals may indeed suffer from a mental illness like a paraphilic disorder. They may also have comorbid psychosis, mood or substance disorders that would be relevant for the court to hear about. There is a general principle in the law that individuals should not be punished for illness. This was highlighted in Powell v. Texas [30] and Robinson v. California [31] where punishing someone for the "status" of being an addict violated the eighth amendment's prohibition against cruel and unusual punishment. However, this did not prohibit punishing illegal behaviors despite recognizing this may not be an effective crime-reducing intervention.

Increased Sentence Length

Sexual offences increasingly carry significant sentences. This is based on legal principles of justice, ensuring what society determines is reasonable punishment for harming others and doing illegal behavior. Further, there is some suggestion that longer sentences may deter others from offending and deter individuals from recidivating. The literature generally does not support these contentions. Few if any offenders contemplate the fact they are doing wrong and will get caught/punished at the time of offending. Further, most sexual offenders are at relatively low risk of sexually re-offending at around 13 % for all untreated sexual offenders [8, 32]. The exception may be for some high-risk offenders who may have decreasing risk as they age [33]. Experts may have a role in educating the court around these issues.

Civil Commitment and Indefinite Sentencing

In theory, standard criminal sentencing interventions should sufficiently protect the public from sexual offenders. However, it has long been recognized that some offenders may be of such high risk that special measures are needed to protect society. This might include pedophiles who recidivate recurrently despite appropriate interventions, sexually motivated psychopaths, and sexually sadistic offenders. Since the inception of these laws, psychiatrists and psychologists have often been a party to these high-stakes hearings, giving diagnostic evaluations, risk assessments, and treatment recommendations to the court. While there are limited numbers of very high risk offenders who may require extraordinary measures to manage their risk, unfortunately many of the laws to deal with these offenders spring out of high profile cases with little evidence for necessity or efficacy. Further, even if based on sound theory, there is a significant potential to distort the intention of these laws.

Sexual psychopath laws had a first wave in the 1930s and 1940s in the United States and Canada [29, 34]. Much like current laws, these laws usually resulted in indefinite sentences or civil commitment of offenders who were deemed highest risk. Chenier notes that many people in this era believed that sexual offences in all forms were a result of mental disorder, particularly those offences of a recurrent nature. For example, some psychiatric testimony dating to 1905 explained that a "disease of the mind" caused "gross indecency" cases of consensual male homosexual acts. Psychiatric testimony was also used in determining which offenders would be deemed sexual psychopaths. While these sexual psychopath laws may have had some valid purpose of containing the highest risk individuals, many instead were crafted to deter morally unacceptable behavior.

In a contemporaneous evaluation of the Canadian law by the Royal Commission [35], it was noted that a person could be declared a dangerous sexual predator for serious sexual offences, including rape and sexual contact with children. However, this also extended to less severe offences including "buggary" (i.e., homosexual intercourse), bestiality, and gross indecency.

American laws were similarly broad and individuals were declared sexual psychopaths for serious offences including sexual assaults and sexual contact with minors. However, there were examples of declaring individuals as sexual psychopaths for less severe offences, including for public masturbation, for an African-American following a Caucasian woman, a non-aggressive homosexual convicted of passing bad checks, exhibitionists, voyeurs, and consenting adult homosexuals [36].

These laws were criticized early on [37]. Either they were abused for use on low risk individuals or alternatively, seldom being used. It was theorized this lack of use was related to several issues. Many laws were developed in an initial "panic" from a high profile case. When the "panic" wore off, no motivation existed to use these. Further, it was recognized at the time that there were no facilities to care for these individuals as state hospitals were already filled with psychotic patients. Courts were also reluctant to view offenders as patients and opted instead for criminal justice interventions. Lastly, offenders were advised to not speak with psychiatrists such that no diagnosis could be made and civil commitment could not occur.

Despite the initial decline and failure of these civil commitment laws, a second wave of legislation started with many states currently having "sexually violent predator laws."

Many of these statutes require the presence of a disorder (defined legally, not medically) combined with ongoing future risk (e.g., see Booth and Schmedlen [38]). These laws have faced a number of legal challenges. In Specht v. Patterson [39], Francis Specht was sentenced under the Colorado Sex Offenders Act to an indefinite sentence without a hearing. He appealed and ultimately the U.S. Supreme Court held that his 14th Amendment right to due process required a formal hearing with reasonable protections such as counsel, cross-examination and the right to testify.

Later, in Allen v. Illinois [40], Terry Allen was convicted of Unlawful Restraint and Deviant Sexual Assault. He underwent a Sexually Dangerous Persons Act evaluation, but later appealed the finding after a psychiatrist disclosed information about him. He suggested that his fifth amendment right against self-incrimination was violated. The U.S. Supreme Court disagreed, noting that as the procedure was a civil hearing (i.e., not a criminal procedure), the same protections were not guaranteed.

In another set of hearings (In re: Young and In re: Cunningham [41]), appeals were launched as both individuals had new sexually violent predator laws applied retrospectively after their initial convictions. The U.S. Supreme Court again held that, as these were civil procedures, the legal principles of *ex post facto* (i.e., having a new law apply retroactively) and *double jeopardy* (i.e., being punished twice for the same offence) did not apply. However, the court did note that as the goal was treatment and not punishment, the least restrictive option should be pursued.

In Kansas v. Hendricks [42], again these arguments were made and the U.S. Supreme Court again denied noting these were civil matters. Further, he argued that he was so restricted that he could not be treated; the court did not see this as problematic. In Seling v. Young [43], similar arguments were made and again rejected. In short, the courts appear to view these laws as constitutionally sound though there may be some protections to ensure an appropriate but lower level of due process and to have treatment as a goal rather than punishment.

In Canada, the legislators have enacted similar laws, though these are criminal sentences rather than civil commitment. Once a conviction is entered, the Attorney General has the option to request a Dangerous Offender designation. This offers either fixed or indefinite sentencing with either fixed or indefinite supervision for those who do leave jail. Again, psychiatrists are integral to the process and give evidence on diagnosis, risk, and management.

Post-release Conditions

When sexual offenders finally do re-enter the community, there are a number of potential legal interventions to manage their risk. Probation or parole conditions will be in place with the idea that such conditions will decrease the risk posed by the offender. This might include reporting to the probation/parole officer, living in approved or supervised accommodations, curfew, avoiding playgrounds, not using the internet, and other restrictions.

It is also required in many jurisdictions that sexual offenders register on release from prison. There may be zoning restrictions preventing offenders from living in certain areas or towns. There has also been a move to have offenders wear global position system devices (GPS) for tracking. While these interventions may provide reassurances to the public, there is little evidence that they are helpful. They may instead put unintentional barriers on attaining stable employment, stable housing, and stable relationship and thus inadvertently increase risk [44–46].

Mental Health Interventions

Beyond external controls, there are a number of mental health interventions for sexual offenders and those with paraphilias. Although high quality research evidence is lacking, likely these interventions do provide some benefit when used appropriately but experienced clinicians.

At times, legal issues also come into play. While interventions may be helpful, at times courts will want to use treatment providers as "police." This may include mandating attendance at group therapy or individual therapy. Unfortunately, this forced psychotherapy is unlikely to be helpful. Further, moving into a strict policing role will decrease the likehood of developing a therapeutic alliance with patients. For example, if an offender is struggling with alcohol/drugs and is occasionally yielding to cravings, they would be unlikely to seek out a "policing therapist's" help for fear of being reprimanded.

Beyond the lack of efficacy of mandated psychological treatment, courts at times will also demand that health care providers give court-ordered treatment. This might include injectable anti-testosterone agents or actual surgical castration. This can put the clinician in a significant ethical and professional dilemma, as true informed consent (free from coercion) cannot be given. Further, ordered treatments may bring significant health risks to the patient that court does not have expertise to weigh. Offenders may also be ordered treatments that pose significant physical risks despite having other sufficient risk management strategies in place.

An exception may exist in the case of those individuals with comorbid serious mental illness who are either okay getting treatment for their underlying illness; or, alternatively, those who are incapable to consent and for whom independent substitute consent has been obtained. Clinicians should remember their primary duty is to follow professional ethics and responsibilities of their profession and not to act as a blind agent of the court.

Clinical Case(s)

Mr. Smith is a 47-year-old man who has a long criminal history:

- At 13 years old—truancy charges and placed in youth facility for 1 month
- At 15 years old—drunk and disorderly charge (dealt with via diversion)

- At 17 years old—conviction for theft × 2
- At 18 years old—possession of child pornography; served 1 year in jail
- At 25 years old—possession of substance (cocaine); served 1 year in jail
- At 30 years old—aggravated assault (on domestic partner); served 3 years in jail with 2 years probation
- At 34 years old—breach of probation, possession of cocaine, armed Robbery—in jail 5 years with 3 years probation
- At 40 years old—sexual interference (fondling 10 year old niece), possession of child pornography—in jail 5 years with 3 years probation

Police have now charged with two additional counts of sexual interference (fondling two neighborhood girls, aged 7 and 10 years old).

The clinician may face numerous legal demands around such a patient. In this case, the Court has requested a Sexually Violent Predator evaluation.

- The first step should be to ensure that the clinician has appropriate skills and expertise to do this type of evaluation. A clarification of the facts should be obtained, including likely awaiting a conviction on the current offences. The legislation and relevant jurisprudence should also be reviewed. A thorough evaluation should then proceed which includes reviewing comprehensive files and then a diagnostic interview and testing of Mr. Smith with informed consent. The clinician should then make a psychiatric diagnosis and complete a risk assessment [47].

Clarification of these issues reveals that Mr. Smith has struggled with intellectual disability throughout his life. His IQ is 48 and he has mainly lived in group homes all of his life. With his charges, it is clear that he has significant impulse control problems and has low frustration tolerance due to limited problem solving. At around the age of 24, he also started to develop auditory hallucinations and delusional ideas of persecution which persist when free of substances. It is clear he likely has schizophrenia which has responded well to treatment, though compliance is problematic.

Phallometric testing shows no arousal to children and instead shows high levels of arousal to consensual adult heterosexual situations. In reviewing the file, it is clear that he has had significant problems fitting in with adults his own age given his mild dysmorphic periods and immaturity. His recent charges at 40 years old and currently occurred when off of his antipsychotic medication. He appears to have a pattern of establishing friendships with younger girls who accept his immaturity, intellectual deficits, and odd appearance.

- At this stage, it should be apparent that, while high risk, Mr. Smith has significant clinical issues contributing to his offending. Many of these are modifiable/dynamic factors. Mr. Smith likely would not be pedophilic based on his negative phallometric testing and offences. The clinician should prepare a comprehensive psycho-legal report aimed at the questions from the court.
- Other legal issues may be:
  - Providing testimony if required, remembering that your duty is to the court to provide fair, objective, and non-partisan opinion evidence and not to decide the outcome of the case
  - Making recommendations for treatment and risk management
  - Providing treatment and follow-up of this individual
  - Exploring the capacity to consent to treatment in an individual with psychosis and intellectual disability, including treatment of any sexual disorders
  - Collaborating with probation/parole and support workers to minimize risk
  - Educating police/parole and law enforcement around stigmatization issues

Recommendations

In working with individuals who have paraphilic disorders and/or have committed sexual offences, clinicians face numerous potential legal issues as outlined. With this it is recommended that:

- Clinicians should be aware of their own skills and knowledge, including limitations which may prevent them working with this complex population
- Clinicians must be aware of the diagnostic criteria for paraphilic disorders, including literature regarding the relationship to offending and risk
- Clinicians should also be knowledgeable regarding the limits of DSM-5 diagnosis and contentions
- Clinicians should be able to educate the court when a paraphilic disorder may be relevant for risk and other court purposes including when paraphilic disorders does not relate to court issues
- Clinicians must navigate the societal and legal influences around sexual behaviors and avoid pathologizing normative sexual behaviors
- Clinicians should ensure ethical practice when facing legal pressures

Acknowledgement

Disclosure Statement

"The author has nothing to disclose."

References

1. Frances A, First MB. Hebephilia is not a mental disorder in DSM-IV-TR and should not become one in DSM-5. J Am Acad Psychiatry Law. 2011;39(1):78–85.
2. Fabian JM. Diagnosing and litigating hebephilia in sexually violent predator civil commitment proceedings. J Am Acad Psychiatry Law. 2011;39(4):496–505.
3. Zonana H. Sexual disorders: new and expanded proposals for the DSM-5—do we need them? J Am Acad Psychiatry Law. 2011;39(2):245–9.
4. Fedoroff JP. Forensic and diagnostic concerns arising from the proposed DSM-5 criteria for sexual paraphilic disorder. J Am Acad Psychiatry Law. 2011;39(2):238–41.
5. First MB. DSM-5 and paraphilic disorders. J Am Acad Psychiatry Law. 2014;42(2):191–201.

6. Davies C. Sexual taboos and social boundaries. Am J Sociol. 1982;87(5):1032–63.
7. Greenland C. Sex law reform in an international perspective: England and Wales and Canada. Bull Am Acad Psychiatry Law. 1983;11(4):309–30.
8. Hanson RK, Bussiere MT. Predicting relapse: a meta-analysis of sexual offender recidivism studies. J Consult Clin Psychol. 1998;66(2):348–62.
9. Kingston DA, Firestone P, Moulden HM, Bradford JM. The utility of the diagnosis of pedophilia: a comparison of various classification procedures. Arch Sex Behav. 2007;36(3):423–36.
10. Marshall WL. Clinical and research limitations in the use of phallometric testing with sexual offenders. Sex Offender Treatment. 2006;1(1):1–19.
11. Marshall WL. Diagnostic problems with sexual offenders. In: Marshall WL, Fernandez YM, Marshall LE, Serran GA, editors. Sexual offender treatment: controversial issues. New York: Wiley; 2006. p. 33–43.
12. Marshall WL, Fernandez YM. Phallometric testing with sexual offenders: limits to its value. Clin Psychol Rev. 2000;20(7):807–22.
13. Eccles A, Marshall WL, Barbaree HE. Differentiating rapists and non-offenders using the rape index. Behav Res Ther. 1994;32(5):539–46.
14. Marshall WL, Kennedy P, Yates P. Issues concerning the reliability and validity of the diagnosis of sexual sadism applied in prison settings. Sex Abuse. 2002;14(4):301–11.
15. Lalumière ML, Quinsey VL, Harris GT, Rice M, Trautrimas C. Are rapists differentially aroused by coercive sex in phallometric assessments? Ann N Y Acad Sci. 2003;989:221–4.
16. Frances A, Wollert R. Sexual sadism: avoiding its misuse in sexually violent predator evaluations. J Am Acad Psychiatry Law. 2012;40(3):409–16.
17. Dietz PE, Hazelwood RR, Warren J. The sexually sadistic criminal and his offenses. Bull Am Acad Psychiatry Law. 1990;18(2):163–78.
18. Warren JI, Hazelwood RR, Dietz PE. The sexually sadistic serial killer. J Forensic Sci. 1996;41(6):970–4.
19. Marshall WL, Hucker SJ. Severe sexual sadism: its features and treatment. In: McAnulty RD, Burnette MM, editors. Sex and sexuality, Sexual deviation and sexual offenses, vol. 3. Westport: Praeger/Greenwood; 2006. p. 227–50.
20. Langstrom N, Seto MC. Exhibitionistic and voyeuristic behavior in a Swedish national population survey. Arch Sex Behav. 2006;35:427–35.

21. Clarke SK, Jeglic EL, Calkins C, Tatar JR. More than a nuisance: the prevalence and consequences of frotteurism and exhibitionism. Sex Abuse. 2016;28(1):3–19.
22. Sharma BR. Disorders of sexual preference and medicolegal issues thereof. Am J Forensic Med Pathol. 2003;24(3):277–82.
23. Abel GG, Osborn C. The paraphilias. The extent and nature of sexually deviant and criminal behavior. Psychiatr Clin North Am. 1992;15(3):675–87.
24. Briken P, Habermann N, Berner W, Hill A. The influence of brain abnormalities on psychosocial development, criminal history and paraphilias in sexual murderers. J Forensic Sci. 2005;50(5):1204–8.
25. Holoyda B, Newman W. Zoophilia and the law: legal responses to a rare paraphilia. J Am Acad Psychiatry Law. 2014;42(4):412–20.
26. Stoneage D. Donkey Love [Film] 2012.
27. Massen J. Zoophilie. Die sexuelle Liebe zu Tieren. Cologne: Pinto Press; 1994.
28. Booth BD, Sorrentino RM, Moore S, Hatters-Friedman SJ. Heavy petting: bestiality and zoophilia. AAPL Newslett. 2015;40(2):24.
29. La Fond JQ. The costs of enacting a sexual predator law. Psychol Pub Pol'y L Mar-Jun. 1998;4(1–2):468–504.
30. Powell v. Texas, 392 U.S. 514 (1968).
31. Robinson v. California, 370 U.S. 660 (1962).
32. Hanson RK, Morton-Bourgon KE. Predictors of sexual recidivism: an updated meta-analysis. Ottawa: Public Safety and Emergency Preparedness Canada; 2004.
33. Hanson RK, Harris AJ, Helmus L, Thornton D. High-risk sex offenders may not be high risk forever. J Interpers Violence. 2014;29(15):2792–813.
34. Chenier E. The criminal sexual psychopath in Canada: sex, psychiatry and the law. Can Bull Med Hist. 2003;20(1):75–101.
35. McRuer JC, Desrochers G, Kinnear H, Worrall J, Martel E, Wake FR. Report of the Royal Commission on the criminal law relating to criminal sexual psychopaths. Ottawa: The Queen's Printer; 1958.
36. Lieb R, Quinsey VL, Berliner L. Sexual predators and social policy. Crime Justice. 1998;23:43–114.
37. Sutherland EH. The sexual psychopath laws. J Crim Law Criminol. 1950;40(5):543–54.
38. Booth BD, Schmedlen G. Sexually violent predator laws. J Am Acad Psychiatry Law. 2006;34(4):553–5.

39. Specht v Patterson, 386 U.S. 605 (1967).
40. Allen v. Illinois, 478 U.S. 364 (1986).
41. In re: Young & Cunningham, 857 P.2d 989 (1993).
42. Kansas v. Hendricks, 521 U.S. 346 (U.S. Supreme Court 1997).
43. Seling v. Young, 531 U.S. 250 (2001).
44. Agan AY. Sex offender registries: fear without function? J Law Econ. 2011;54(1):207–39.
45. Prescott JJ, Rockoff JE. Do sex offender registration and notification laws affect criminal behavior? J Law Econ. 2011;54(1):161–206.
46. Barton RA, Wesley RW, Spillane SR. Special review: assessment of electronic monitoring of sex offenders on parole and the impact of residency restrictions. California: State of California; 2014.
47. Bradford JM, Seto MC, Booth BD. Forensic assessment of sex offenders. In: Simon RI, Gold LH, editors. The American Psychiatric Publishing textbook of forensic psychiatry. 2nd ed. Washington, DC: American Psychiatric Association Press; 2010.

Chapter 18
Cultural Aspects of Unusual Sexual Interests

A. Pacheco Palha and Mário F. Lourenço

Introduction

Unusual sexual interests and paraphilia behaviours are more common than people believe and are known since ancient times. Even in certain historical times and cultures, some were common practice, whilst others belonged to each individual's private sphere. It is from the publication of books by Marquis de Sade that perversions beyond the scope of the bedroom became a subject matter for philosophers and scientists. We know from Freud that we start being such when polymorphous perversion was not exempted from the evil essence of our fundamental fantasies. Perhaps we can finally understand the difficulties of dealing with this concept which, throughout time and the interests of science, turned out to be excluded from the psychiatric glossary.

The name paraphilia does figure in the Mental and Behavioural Disorders ICD-10 Classification, edited by the

A.P. Palha, M.D., Ph.D. (✉)
Faculty of Medicine of Porto University, Rua do Carvalho, 109-4 EA, Porto, Portugal
e-mail: apalha@sapo.pt

M.F. Lourenço, M.D., Ph.D.
Couple's Clinic, Psychiatric and Mental Health Department, Alto Ave Hospital Center, Guimarães, Portugal

R. Balon (ed.), *Practical Guide to Paraphilia and Paraphilic Disorders*, DOI 10.1007/978-3-319-42650-1_18

World Health Organization under F 65 (part of adult personality disorders…) [1]. That part is called disorders of sexual preference, including paraphilia. In DSM-IV Classification, we have an entry that explains that Psychiatry has replaced the term "perversion" with the term "paraphilia," due to the pejorative weight that the former concept has in common sense soften the stigma that such word puts in our normal "human sexuality" leaving it just for legal use [2]. In DSM-5 there is a section on Paraphilia Disorders (302) [1, 2]. In DSM-5 there is a section on Paraphilia Disorders (302) [54].

In this chapter we would like to outline the reflection of how cultural aspects are intrinsically connected to paraphilia. The discourse on sexuality appears in certain socio-historical moments as an attempt to regulate sexual practice according to the standards of the time. In this perspective, it is understood that social and political control of human behaviour can only be achieved through control of the body and sexuality, being sexuality a construction inseparable from the discourse on power within such is established [3].

In a simplistic way, it is possible to state that human societies control human sexual activity given that this is responsible for the reproduction of our species. The taboo acts psychologically, from the identification of the features that make the forbidden object to be consumed [4, 5].

A culture is an abstract description of trends towards word uniformity and artefacts of a human group. Sexuality is a highly cultural-dependent construct, although there are still just a few researches on relationships [6].

It is almost certain that all human societies throughout history have imposed boundaries or limits on all types of sexual behaviours which are considered acceptable. Some societies support male dominance over women, whilst some might be conservative when discussing their sexual problems [7].

Interestingly, there is some tendency for people to act as if the sexual norms of each time and culture were the only correct ones, and therefore they tend to appear intolerant to those who do not share their view. Thus, we understand, for example, that sex with animals can be tolerated in some cultures, whilst in others a simple masturbation act is punishable by death. It is true that Western society became more permissive regarding sexuality after World War II but, even today, there are very good people who still think that masturbating is normal and acceptable in adolescence and youth, but only if that practice is performed with moderation! [8–10]

But especially in the Western world, throughout history, aphorism has always prevailed: "Public virtues and private vices." Only through this supreme duality is it possible to understand the sexual excesses of some figures in Western history, as it is the case of Theodora, wife of the Roman Emperor Justinian, where even by today's standards she would be considered strange and surely perverse. It is said that Theodora used to complain about God only giving her three holes in her body.

The term paraphilia was coined in 1922 by Wilhelm Stekel and it is a combination of the words "para," meaning beyond the usual, and "philia," meaning love [11, 12].

But historically, paraphilia was termed as perversion. Sexual deviance is a topic that captivates the media's attention and causes widespread apprehension both inside the criminal justice system and within the general public, although clinical experience shows that the formation of paraphilia does not certainly lead to dysfunctional behaviours, but it depends on the situations being harmful or not [13–15].

Simply having paraphilia is, obviously, not illegal. Acting in response to paraphilic urges, however, may be illegal, and in some cases subjects the paraphilic person to severe sanctions [16].

Science and Culture: A Complex Dialogue

Sexuality couldn't exist in the culture without words, images, metaphors and symbols to represent it [17].

Complexity makes the sexual experience a unique and original reality for all human activities, but at the same time it also reveals its weakness from a scientific perspective, as it removes the possibility of being an objective and quantifiable reality.

Sexual activities often function as signifiers for personal and social idiosyncrasies to which they have no intrinsic connection, which applies to issues of power, the power in society and power in gender relations. Most all, in the complex human society, in general, the ethnic and religious background of the individual emphasizes male dominance and control over female sexuality versus those that reward the opposite view [18].

Except for sexual masochism, where the sex ratio is estimated to be 20 males for each female, other paraphilia cases are almost never diagnosed to females, although some have been reported [19].

It is easy to see that much perversion of the past is currently supported or at least considered as less perverse behaviours. At the same time, some of the old customs, sometimes rogue at the time, are now seen as horrendous acts. Probably more than in another historical period, currently we are able to understand the intricate relationships established between human sexuality and cultural influences. However, there are still difficulties in bringing science closer to culture. However, the role and development of paraphilia across cultures varies, with cultures defining what is legal or illegal. Such differences make collection of paraphilia epidemiological data and comparisons a problematic issue. This discussion suggests that cultural characteristics may influence the rate of reported paraphilia, as well as the rate of paraphilia itself [20].

When comes the time to seek treatment, cultural variables hamper the orientation and approach to paraphilic patients. In an Asian cultural context, not only do individuals suffering from sexual disorders that include paraphilic ones might feel uncomfortable when visiting clinic, but also do the medical personnel when treating patients [6]. Asian patients might feel extreme anxiety or insecurity when exposed to sexual materials in front of practitioners, given the fact that they already feel uncomfortable consulting healthcare professionals regarding their sexual problems. Alternative medicine, however, is extremely common in Asia for treating sexual disorders, including non-prescription hormones and physical treatment like vacuum devices [6]. Studies found that Asian men feel more comfortable using traditional medicine because it is cheaper than western medicine and is more identifiable with their values and beliefs [6]. Exposing intimate life to a stranger, even if to a health professional, always causes a high dose of embarrassment, which increases remarkably when revealing tastes or sexual preferences that are not accepted by others. In this sense, unfortunately, culture is the "major barrier across processes of assessment, treatment and reintegration with [sic] offenders [21]."

Knowing the importance of sociocultural influences in atypical sexual behaviour was expected in a scientific approach that could impose up to other models of paraphilia analysis. Traditional studies of paraphilics are based on psychiatric and forensic populations. The vast majority of these populations suffer from isolated minority syndrome to various extents. This has created a not very positive image about this population in the psychiatric literature. Sociological studies based on populations from sexual minority organizations give a totally different image and perhaps this is one of the different approaches missing in medicine today [22–24].

Most likely, awareness of different cultural patterns has been used to reinforce this idea rather than to confront our own culture-bound conceptions.

Obscurantism and Moral Repression

It does not seem easy to venture into the historical and cultural understanding of sexual perversion without having a clear concept of what is precisely sought, the historical evolution of one of the most used criteria in observing cultural changes made on the concept of perversion methods.

Paraphilic behaviours have been present in all human societies throughout different historical moments. With the differentiation of primates and the emergence of *Homo sapiens*, the need for a level of social organization and establishment of normative rules for the relationship of individuals became necessary. Within this increasingly complex social organization, rules were inevitably emerging to regulate the various aspects of individual activities, including sexual ones [25].

So, even when possessed by intense sexual desire, the male came to power only to practice intercourse with a female under certain conditions, also imposed when the situation was reversed. This has created a whole complex of ritual symbolism—which ended in marriage, as we know it—to standardize what is socially acceptable in terms of exercising sexuality. Due to primitive cultures, our current view of human experience is not more evolved as they were more "natural" or less "civilized" in the use of their bodies. These cultures had different prohibitions and obligations were always linked to belief systems and magic. Sexuality was inseparable from economic activities, social relations, symbolic systems and mythical representations. Every human society has its own conception of what life and interpersonal relationships are, taken from experience and moral convictions, which are characteristic of members of a particular human group. The further back we go in time, the more difficult it is to distinguish normal from abnormal. Certain practices, such as homosexuality and masturbation were considered Paraphilic, though now are considered normal and acceptable variations of sexual activity. But historical evidence shows that, in particular, sexual relations between persons of the same sex have always existed in all cultures. Indeed, the first reports on that appeared around the third Egyptian dynasty, about 2500 years BC [26].

Certain periods of autocratic policies have reinforced the rigidity of sexual morals, as it happened during the long period of Salazar Dictatorship, namely regarding women status [27].

In some ancient civilizations, homosexual practices, especially among adult men and young ones, were repudiated only when they threatened to subvert social hierarchy [28].

A person unrelated to modern Western culture does not recognize the word sexuality or associates that word to the kind of experiences we know today. For example, it is clear that sexual practices of the Sambia tribe of Papua New Guinea are unacceptable to Western sexual culture. Among other things, men learn to perform fellatio (oral sex) before adolescence. The goal is to only eat the sperm, which grants protective properties, in order to store sufficient quantities to inseminate women after puberty. Once they have their first child, this ritualized homosexuality disappears completely [29, 30]. We also know that many African tribes do not condemn masturbation practiced alone or in groups, behaviour that always scandalized many of the white colonizers [31]. Herodotus, Pindar, and Plutarch wrote of sacred congress with goats in ancient Egypt; African and the Chinese are all reported to have tolerated some bestiality in the past, mostly by men [31]. Sadomasochistic topics go through the history of mankind, with associated descriptions Dionysian rites to eighteenth-century British flagellation brothels until some carnal expiation practices of Catholics [32, 33].

Throughout time in the Western world, non-consensual sexual practices have been opposed by religious powers. Let it be said in support of the truth that social rejection of a given behaviour is above all moral rejections. Clearly, sexual perversion has strong religious roots, like so many things, and extends to each society that privatizes those beliefs. Many ideas and concepts lose their collective strength that they previously had. With Christianity, sexuality comes as a matter related to customs that shall be regulated by an external source to the subject. In fact, sexual practices were governed by three major codes: Canon Law, Christian Ministry and Civil Law. In the Christian era, paraphilics were persecuted by the Inquisition and condemned its practitioners to death. Humanitarian law of the Old Testament said: "Anyone who cohabits with a beast dies." [34] This compliance is illustrated in the following passage: "In July 1659, a (Spanish) gardener was throwing garbage with a little donkey, took him from the field to the orchard and fell in love with this beast, taking advantage of it at noon. He was seen and fled, but him and the love of his donkey Maron were caught in Alcalá [35]."

There is a direct relation between the development of Christian conceptions of sexuality and the age of obscurantism that prevailed in the middle age. The middle age: a gap in human development? It can be said that the middle age remained and deepened the negative view of sexuality. Moreover, it is now considered as something that shames the human being's sexual desire, identified with something that is bad by itself. The middle age, in the direct heritage of thought of Plato and Aristotle, defends the dualistic conception of the soul and body with the corresponding depreciation of the latter; it still does not recognize any connection between love and sex and defines love in purely spiritual terms. Knowing the middle Ages, that vision bequeathed to sexuality, there was nothing better than to see the two theologians/medieval philosophers who enjoyed greater prestige in the Christian world: Augustine and Thomas d'Aquin [36].

Augustine, who was the most influential theologian of the Middle Age and which is still accepted as a higher authority in matters of doctrine, taught that the body is corrupted by original sin; He expressed great shame for the youth's sexual activities; He argued that all love must be God's love and lust is bad. A reasonable person would prefer procreation to be achieved without sexual lust; sex served only for procreation, and even legitimate marital relations were accompanied by shame, which, he said, is indicted for privacy where the relationship takes place [37–39].

By placing the origin of evil in sexuality, i.e. "sexualizing" the original sin, Augustine left his greatest legacy to Christian morality: lust was the original sin; man is the result of sin. This design made the world somewhat hindered by the demands of the body that prevented access of the soul; the human being became fragile and blamed by desire, which led to an unprecedented exaltation of virginity. Moreover, the sexualized view of original sin makes man a helpless victim of an unscrupulous and unprincipled woman who seduces him, causing him to sin; and this sin is always sexual. Hence arises the negative image of women, still present in the Western view as responsible for the fall; on the other hand, man appears as a spiritual being in its origin, a helpless victim of a diabolical woman. St. Thomas d'Aquin (1225–1274) was one of the biggest contributors to the establishment of a sexual ideology that deals in a negative view with sexual issues and led to discrimination against certain sexual behaviours. The Thomist principle of sin argues that nature was created and ordained by God and as such cannot be contradicted by human behaviour. Applying these concepts to the specific field of sexuality, it is understood that St. Thomas d'Aquin and all his followers believed that sexual intercourse only served for reproduction of the human species: the sperm should only be deposited in a natural vain (the vagina). If the semen was deposited elsewhere than the vagina it was considered unnatural and unacceptable. The reproduction of the species is the cause of sex and not the other way around. Who then does not do this is perverted, inverted and abnormal [40–43].

The Medicalization of Sexual Deviance

If there is a stigma attached to sexual conduct, it is paraphilia. Tagged by perversion, deviation or aberration, rejected by society and sometimes despised by it, paraphilics have come a long way in being recognized as sufferers by psychiatric nosological classifications. The stigmatizing of what is outside the ordinary mortals and generating social isolation and moralistic attitudes also aims to express what medical diagnosis have ended up trying to do, i.e. an arrangement in supposedly normal categories. The abnormality criteria are changing according to the historical moment. Therefore, the various areas of scientific knowledge have serious difficulties in establishing diagnosing criteria and therapeutic manuals. In mid-last century, the dissemination of psychoanalysis perversion became an inevitable traveling companion, and therefore scientific publications reduced the noise produced about it in the previous two centuries [44].

At least in some situations the paraphilic is no longer seen as a diabolical figure that frightens most people, that will destroy families and misrepresent social customs. Good sense begins to prevail as all paraphilic are not considered dangerous mentally ill. Three closely related sources for a scientific awareness of sexual variability can be pinpointed: first, the pioneering work of nineteenth century sexologists such as Magnus Hirschfeld and others, whose labelling and categorizing led them outside their own culture; second, Freud's writings, providing a breath of fresh air to thought and Western culture; and third, the work of anthropologists who attempted to chart varieties of sexual behaviour and who supplied the data on which sexologists relied on [45].

Doctors are increasingly medicalising and pathologising sexual and gender deviance. More than an arrogant manifest or statement of a militant approach, this expression reveals a reality that has been worrying many people. Foucault was one of the first to draw attention to the presence of ideology in medical discourse on issues related to sexuality. Foucault's *History of Sexuality* is based on his view that discursive practices in the medical community created deviant identities and produced and regulated sex practices that started in late nineteenth century [3].

The clinical follow-up has proved that people associated with paraphilic behaviours are in fact the complex subject of analysis of the loupe of Medicine. Every person with paraphilia can be unintelligible from a strictly physiological point of view, but intelligible when considering the whole culture.

In this sense, you do not have to necessarily be mentally disordered in some way to be attracted to someone who falls outside of a particular ideal of human figure. All the controversies surrounding the DSM-5 conceptualization reveal to what extent problems associated with an unusual sexual interest can be primarily sexual, whilst in other cases they are related to another mental disorder, or are social disorders rather than psychiatric ones [46].

Conclusion

Sex as we know it was invented in the eighteenth century, with the production of a binary gender system. The notion of "normal" and "natural" gender distinctions continued throughout the nineteenth century, given that the middle class family was a central organizing principle for society [47].

It has been widely recognized for almost a century that attitudes towards paraphilic behaviour are culturally specific, and have varied enormously across different cultures and throughout various historical periods. Despite the variability that a cultural criterion introduces in the analysis of the phenomenon of paraphilia, what is certain is that these sexual behaviours cause damage and suffering: inciting to obligatory rituals; entailing sexual dysfunction and legal or social complications; requiring the participation of individuals without their consent. This instrumentation/dehumanization of the other implies not taking into account one's will and one's desire. In fact, the more the paraphilic diverts another from its normal practice, the more rewarding the act becomes for him. Thus, sexuality is a solitary act, mostly a masturbatory one since the incapacity to experience intimacy; there is no connection with the other. As it turns out, there are tenuous boundaries between paraphilia and offense, compulsiveness and sexual violence. Note that not all paraphilia corresponds to illegal or criminal acts and, on the other hand, not all sexual offenses are linked to the existence of paraphilia. For example, rape is not identified as paraphilia, but in the course of this offensive act, there may be behaviours that are identified as being paraphilia.

Such is the burden that cultural and religious affairs have to atypical sexual behaviour that this has caused some exaggerations in the opposite direction. To some extent, Kinsey contributed to this confusion in his efforts to ban the moral assessment of sexual behaviours, trying to replace it by dispassionate scientific reflection. In doing so, he eventually and excessively extended the concept of normality to include many behaviours that are considered increasingly beyond all limits. Kinsey suggested that what was common and normal among other mammals was, from this evidence, biologically and psychologically normal in humans [48].

By introducing the variable culture in the discussion of the pathogenesis and the definition of atypical behaviours, we take a risk by using it to provide evidence for or against paraphilia's naturalness. In line with a certain purifying vision of what is bizarre, most of the more elaborate science-minded commentaries seemed to reduce "cultures" to places where the natural substrate of "no normative erotic orientation" may or may not be attested. But culture defines and culture causes paraphilia, this is the key to understanding sexuality [49]. Likewise is the culture that shapes gender and is present in different stages of the human life cycle [50]. Only then we can understand that Homosexuality and masturbation are rare or nonexistent in two African cultures: the Aka and Ngandu, not because they are frowned upon or punished, but because they are not part of the cultural models of sexuality in either ethnic group [49, 50]. Only then we can understand that Homosexuality and masturbation are rare or nonexistent in two African cultures: the Aka and Ngandu, not because they are frowned upon or punished, but because they are not part of the cultural models of sexuality in either ethnic group [52].

Cultural variables enhance religious beliefs, as in the case of Hinduism. Hinduism does not condemn bestiality in certain circumstances or masturbation According to this religion, seeking Kama (sensual pleasures) is one of the four objectives of human life. However, celibacy (Brahmacharya) is one of the foundations of Hinduism and masturbation is one of the impediments to purity during the Brahmacharya phase of the life [51].

It is relevant to stress that cultures issues have been discussed deeply during the process of writing the DSM-5. Unfortunately the sexual behaviour was not contemplated with such interest.

We, as a society, love to make things about sex and make sex problematic; after all, we never learn from past mistakes.

References

1. World Health Organization. CID-10, Portuguese version—translation of the WHO Collaborator Center to the classification of Diseases in Portuguese. 9th ed., rev. São Paulo: EDUSP; 2003.
2. American Psychiatric Association. DSM-IV-TR: manual of diagnostic and statistics of mental disorders. 4th ed. Lisbon: Climepsi; 2002.

3. Foucault M. The use of pleasure: the history of sexuality, vol. 2. New York: Vintage; 1985.
4. Rubin G. The "political economy" of sex. In: Feminist Anthropology: a reader. Oxford: Blackwell; 2009. p. 87.
5. Allan K, Burridge K. Forbidden words: taboo and the censoring of language. Cambridge: Cambridge University Press; 2006.
6. Kalra G, Tandon A, Rao TS. Sexual disorders in Asians: a review. Asian J Psychiatry. 2014;7:80–2.
7. Davies C. Sexual taboos and social boundaries. Am J Sociol. 1982;87:1032–63.
8. Broude GJ. Extramarital sex norms in cross-cultural perspective. Cross-Cult Res. 1980;15(3):181–218.
9. Herek GM. Beyond "homophobia": thinking about sexual prejudice and stigma in the twenty-first century. Sex Res Soc Policy. 2004;1(2):6–24.
10. Wight D, Plummer ML, Mshana G, Wamoyi J, Shigongo ZS, Ross DA. Contradictory sexual norms and expectations for young people in rural Northern Tanzania. Soc Sci Med. 2006;62(4):987–97.
11. Stekel W. Sexual aberrations: the phenomena of fetishism in relation to sex. New York: Liveright Pub. Corp; 1930.
12. Firestone P, Dozois DJA. Abnormal psychology perspectives. 3rd ed. Toronto: Pearson Prentice Hall; 2007.
13. Money J. Response: paraphilia defined. Harv Rev Psychiatry. 1994;2(1):41–2.
14. First MB. DSM-5 proposals for paraphilias: suggestions for reducing false positives related to use of behavioral manifestations. Arch Sex Behav. 2010;39(6):1239–44.
15. Hamilton M. Adjudicating sex crimes as mental disease. Pace Law Rev. 2013;33:536–99.
16. Malin HM, Saleh FM. Paraphilia's: clinical and forensic considerations. Psychiatric Times. 2007;24(5):1–4.
17. Porter R, Hall L. The facts of life: the creation of sexual knowledge in Britain, 1650–1950. New Haven: Yale University Press; 1995.
18. Paniagua FA. Culture-bound syndromes, cultural variations, and psychopathology. In: Cuellar J, Paniagua FA, editors. Handbook of multicultural mental health: assessment and treatment of diverse populations. New York: Academic Press; 2000. p. 139–69.
19. Beier KM. Female analogies to perversion. J Sex Marital Ther. 2000;26(1):79–93.

20. Bhugra D, Popelyuk D, McMullen I. Paraphilia's across cultures: contexts and controversies. J Sex Res. 2010;47(2–3):242–56.
21. Tamatea AJ, Webb M, Boer DP. The role of culture in sexual offender rehabilitation: a New Zealand perspective. In: Boer DP, Eher R, Craig LA, Miner MH, Pfäfflin F, editors. International perspectives on the assessment and treatment of sexual offenders: theory, practice, and research. Chichester: Wiley-Blackwell/ Wiley; 2011. p. 313–30.
22. Fog A. Klinisk bias ved forskning i sexuelle afvigelser. Nordisk Sexologi. 1990;8(2):163–7.
23. Sagarin E. Sex research and sociology: retrospective and prospective. In: Henslin JM, Sagarin E, editors. The sociology of sex. New York: Schocken Books; 1978.
24. Howard JF. Sex variant women in literature: a historical and quantitative survey. New York: Vantage Press; 1956.
25. Fehr E, Fischbacher U. Social norms and human cooperation. Trends Cogn Sci. 2004;8(4):185–90.
26. Miranda, S. de A. Amor entre mulheres: um estudo sócioantropológico das relações afetivas entre pessoas do sexo feminino. Monografia de Graduação, Universidade de Fortaleza, Fortaleza. Recuperado em 11 de abril, 2006, de. 2001. http://www.armariox.com.br/conteudos/cienciaepesquisa.php.
27. Palha AP. (2011). La Sexualidad en tiempo de Salazar. Text presented in the 2014 World Congress of WPA in Madrid.
28. Lacerda M, Pereira C, Camino L. A study about the ways of prejudice against homosexuals in the perspective of social representations. Psicologia. 2002;15(1):165–78.
29. Franke KM. Putting sex to work. Denv UL Rev. 1997;75:1139.
30. Joyce A. Rosemary—ancient bodies, ancient lives, Sex, gender, and archaeology. London: Thames & Hudson; 2008.
31. Staples R. Exploring black sexuality. Lanham: Rowman & Littlefield; 2006.
32. Freeman E. Turn the beat around: Sadomasochism, temporality, history. Differences. 2008;19(1):32–70.
33. Moser C. Sadomasochism. J Soc Work Human Sex. 1989;7(1):43–56.
34. Exodus 22:19. *Holy Bilble*. Sociedad Bíblica Argentina, Buenos Aires, Rosario, Córdoba. Reina Valera 1995.
35. Deleito y Piñuela J. El desenfreno erótico. Madrid: Editorial Alianza; 1995.
36. Soble A, editor. Sex from Plato to Paglia: MZ, vol. 2. London: Greenwood Publishing Group; 2006.

37. O'Meara JJ. Virgil and saint Augustine. The Roman background to Christian sexuality. Augustinus. 1968;13:307–26.
38. Clark EA. St. Augustine on marriage and sexuality, vol. 1. Washington, DC: CUA Press; 1996.
39. Meilaender G. Sweet necessities: food, sex, and saint Augustine. J Relig Ethics. 2001;29(1):3–18.
40. d'Aquin T. Summa theologicae. Nuremberg: Anton Koberger; 1864.
41. Guevin BM. Aquinas's use of Ulpian and the question of physicalism reexamined. Thomist. 1999;63(4):613–28.
42. Rocca GP. Speaking the incomprehensible God: Thomas Aquinas on the interplay of positive and negative theology. Washington, DC: CUA Press; 2004.
43. Kainz H. Human nature and Aquinas' taxonomy of sexual sins. In: Crisis magazine in. 2012. http://www.crisismagazine.com/2012/human-nature-and-aquinas-taxonomy-of-sexual-sins.
44. Roudinesco E. Nuestro lado oscuro. Una historia de los perversos. Barcelona: Anagrama; 2009.
45. Weeks J. Discourse, desire and sexual deviance: some problems in a history of homosexuality. In: Section I: Culture, Society and Sexuality, Part 1: Conceptual Frameworks. New York: Routledge; 1999. p. 119.
46. Moser C. When is an unusual sexual interest a mental disorder? Arch Sex Behav. 2009;38(3):323–5.
47. Laqueur T. Making sex: body and gender from the Greeks to Freud. Boston: Harvard University Press; 1999. p. 149.
48. Kinsey AC, Pomeroy WB, Martin CE. Sexual behavior in the human male. Philadelphia: W.B. Saunders; 1948.
49. Janssen DF. Paraphilia: a cultural or anti-anthropological? Sex Offender Treatment. 2014;9(2).
50. Hewlett BL, Hewlett BS. Hunter-Gatherer adolescence. In: Hewlett BL, editor. Adolescent Identity: evolutionary, cultural and developmental perspectives, vol. 7. New York: Routledge; 2012. p. 73.
51. Johnson WJ. The chaste and celibate state of a student of the Veda. Oxford: Oxford Dictionary of Hinduism, Oxford University Press; 2009.
52. Hewlett BS, Hewlett BL. Sex and searching for children among Aka foragers and Ngandu farmers of Central Africa. Afr Study Monogr. 2010;31:107–25.
53. Dubois-Desaulle G. Bestiality: an historical, medical, legal and literary Study. New York: Priv. print. at the Panurge Press; 1933.
54. American Psychiatric Association. DSM-V: manual of diagnostic and statistics of mental disorders. Washington, DC: American Psychiatric Association; 2013.

Index

R. Balon (ed.), *Practical Guide to Paraphilia and Paraphilic Disorders*, DOI 10.1007/978-3-319-42650-1

MIX
Papier aus verantwortungsvollen Quellen
Paper from responsible sources
FSC® C105338

If you have any concerns about our products,
you can contact us on
ProductSafety@springernature.com

In case Publisher is established outside the EU,
the EU authorized representative is:
Springer Nature Customer Service Center GmbH
Europaplatz 3, 69115 Heidelberg, Germany

Printed by Libri Plureos GmbH
in Hamburg, Germany